‖ SWEETNESS IN THE BLOOD ‖

Sweetness in the Blood

RACE, RISK, AND TYPE 2 DIABETES

James Doucet-Battle

 University of Minnesota Press
Minneapolis
London

This project was supported in part by funding from the University of California Presidential Faculty Research Fellowships in the Humanities, MR-15-328710.

The University of Minnesota Press gratefully acknowledges the financial support provided for the publication of this book by the University of California Office of the President Multi-Campus Research Programs and Initiative Funding, and the UC Humanities Research Institute.

Portions of chapter 1 were originally published as "Ennobling the Neanderthal: Racialized Texts and Genomic Admixture," *Kalfou: A Journal of Comparative and Relational Ethnic Studies* 5, no. 1 (2018): 61–67. Portions of chapters 1, 5, and 6 were originally published as "Bioethical Matriarchy: Race, Gender, and the Gift in Genomic Research," in "Nothing/More: Black Studies and Feminist Technoscience," a special issue of *Catalyst: Feminism, Theory, Technoscience* 2, no. 2 (2016): 1–28. Portions of chapter 4 and 6 were originally published as "Sweet Salvation: One Black Church, Diabetes Outreach, and Trust," *Transforming Anthropology* 24, no. 2 (2016): 125–35.

Published by the University of Minnesota Press
111 Third Avenue South, Suite 290
Minneapolis, MN 55401–2520
http://www.upress.umn.edu

ISBN 978-1-5179-0848-5 (hc)
ISBN 978-1-5179-0849-2 (pb)
Library of Congress record available at https://lccn.loc.gov/2020055823.

The University of Minnesota is an equal-opportunity educator and employer.

To my mother, Clara Doucet, born in the Land of Sugar, Bayou Têche, Louisiana;

My first cultural anthropology professor, a translational bridge between an Afro-French Creole past and the African American reality;

And to my father, James Battle, born on Tobacco Road, Rocky Mount, North Carolina, who should have preceded me in scholarship, but Jim Crow had other demands.

Contents

Abbreviations

AACE/ACE	American Association of Clinical Endocrinologists/American College of Endocrinology
ACC	American College of Cardiology
ACCORD	Action to Control Cardiovascular Risk in Diabetes
ACP	American College of Physicians
ADA	American Diabetes Association
ADCES	Association of Diabetes Care and Education Specialists, formerly American Association of Diabetes Educators (**AADE**)
ADVANCE	Action in Diabetes and Vascular Disease—Preterax and Diamicron Modified Release Controlled Evaluation
AHA	American Heart Association
AROC	area under the receiver operating characteristic curve
BMI	body mass index
CBE	Center for BioEntrepreneurship (University of California, San Francisco)
CC	cultural competence (training)/cultural competency
CDC	Centers for Disease Control
CDE	certified diabetes educator
CEE	collaborative event ethnography
CHW	community health worker
CRC	Clinical Research Center (a pseudonym)
CRO	clinical research organization
CTSA	Center for Translational Science Awards (National Institutes of Health)

CTSI	Clinical and Translational Science Institute (University of California, San Francisco, School of Medicine)
CVD	cardiovascular disease
dbGaP	Database of Genotype and Phenotype
DPP	Diabetes Prevention Program
DRS	Diabetes Risk Score (Tethys BioSciences PreDX™)
FDA	Food and Drug Administration
GWAS	Genome-Wide Association Studies
Hb	hemoglobin
HbA1c	hemoglobin A1c
IEEE	Institute of Electrical and Electronics Engineers
IGT	impaired glucose tolerance
IOM	Institute of Medicine
IP	intellectual property
IPO	initial public offering
LALES	Los Angeles Latino Eye Study
MetS	(cardio)metabolic syndrome
mtDNA	mitochondrial DNA
NHGRI	National Human Genome Research Institute
NHLBI	National Heart, Lung, and Blood Institute
NIH	National Institutes of Health
OGTT	oral glucose tolerance test
PCRM	Physicians Committee for Responsible Medicine
PRS	polygenic risk scores
ROI	return on investment
S&TS	science and technology studies
SPIE	International Society for Optics and Photonics
ST&S	science, technology, and society
T1D	Type 1 diabetes
T2D	Type 2 diabetes
UCSF	University of California, San Francisco
UGDP	University Group Diabetes Program
VADT	Veterans Affairs Diabetes Trial

Introduction
Sugar's Racial Project
FROM SLAVERY TO DIABETES

> The track sugar has left in modern history is one involving
> masses of people and resources, thrown into productive
> combination by social, economic, and political forces that
> were actively remaking the world.
>
> —Sidney Mintz, *Sweetness and Power*

My maternal grandmother worked in the sugarcane fields of South-western Louisiana during her first four decades of life and lived as a diabetic for her last three decades on earth. I am a part of an Afro-French Creole family from New Iberia, Bayou Têche, deep in rural southwest Louisiana. Fort Attakapas, established in 1769, cemented French colonial rule over a territory occupied by opportunistic colonists from France and later by desperate refugees from Nova Scotia. Slavery was introduced to Louisiana in 1735, nearly a century after its establishment in the French West Indies. The majority of these enslaved Africans were brought from Senegambia by decree of the French Crown, due to their expertise in growing rice, with which the French hoped to feed their slaves in more profitable extractive colonies such as Saint-Domingue (now Haiti) and Martinique.[1]

Despite these ambitious plans, slavery in the Louisiana Colony during French rule barely rose above a domestic form of the institution, with the average household having one or two slaves.[2] The colony did not prove profitable to the French, who found themselves occupied with a troublesome and costly insurrection in Saint-Domingue from 1791–1804. In the face of mounting losses on the battlefield and to the government purse, France ceded the Louisiana Territory to the United States in 1803. The subsequent political, religious, and ideological shifts facilitated the spread of the comparatively more brutal, productive, and profitable Anglo-American form of slavery westward and southward to the Gulf of Mexico. After the Haitian Revolution, more refugees from the island settled in Bayou Têche (specifically the area around St. Martinville) than anywhere else outside of New Orleans. It was a refugee population consisting of white plantation owners, their slaves, and free people of color (*gens du couleur libre*). Their extensive knowledge of sugarcane cultivation contributed to the successful breeding of several varieties of Haitian sugarcane that could withstand the infrequent but devastating cold snaps that descend upon subtropical southern Louisiana. The U.S. sugar industry was born.

Yellow fever epidemics ravaged the area repeatedly throughout the eighteenth and nineteenth centuries.[3] The slow development of industrial-scale slavery in southern Louisiana characterized the precarity of life in the area and highlights the contributions of African, Native American, and Caribbean knowledge bases in fostering the health of what was essentially a subsistence economy. To illustrate the collective memory of these periods of bio-insecurity—and present an example more deserving of historical attention—I quote from a plaque in *le carré*, or town square, outside the Iberia Parish Library that pays homage to Félicité,

> A black woman, native of Haiti. During the yellow fever epidemic here in 1839, she nursed the sick, administered to the dying, closed the eyes of the dead, and wept over their graves. Loved and honored by townspeople for the remainder of her life, she died in January 1852. The day of her burial, every business in New Iberia closed its doors, and every man, woman, and child in town followed her to her last resting place in St. Peter's Cemetery. She was an angel of mercy in a time of pestilence. Her name shall not be allowed to drop into oblivion.

It's not your typical antebellum Southern narrative. The plaque gives an idea of the social nature of the area and its historical ties to the Caribbean. The largest city in Bayou Têche, New Iberia, founded by the Spanish in 1779, was slower than most parts of Louisiana to adopt Anglo-American racial discourses, categories, and exclusionary practices. From the Anglo-redefined racial history of southwestern Louisiana my maternal family emerged: generations of the enslaved, sugarcane farmers, sharecroppers, and plantation owners. Sugar production formed an organizational axis around kinship, labor, consumption, language, and religion as part of an ongoing, contested engagement with labor, history, and the material.[4]

But Félicité's memorial makes no facile claim to tolerant cultural self-congratulation. The brief story of Félicité and the honor accorded her during a period of brutal chattel slavery betrays her relative historical anonymity, one that exposes the sacrificial labor of blackness in supporting the flourishing of white life. The narrative exemplifies an unfulfilled epistemic void and ontological yearning enabled by erasures of black ancestries from the archives. Saidiya Hartman's notion of "Mother loss" diagnoses the historical amnesia concerning Félicité.[5] We do not know Félicité's last name. We do not know whether she had siblings or children, or even descendants still living in the area. She came and went, "an angel of mercy in a time of pestilence," before returning to heaven. On a panel erected beside the bayou, her story is told, from beginning to end, encapsulated in a single paragraph and sealed hermetically against genealogical coherence, *fait ça fait*. The recurrent grafting of the white settler-colonist onto the bare rootstock of semi-anonymous black labor in producing better fruits for all, or for our purposes, *sweetness,* furnishes a visual template I suggest the reader may find generative throughout this book.

SUGAR, SLAVERY, AND DIABETES

As a child born and raised in New York, I experienced this often-disconcerting familial past during our family trips down to the land of sugar. We traveled by car to New Iberia, where we stayed with my Tantie (Auntie) Francine, a very large woman with two very large daughters, my favorite cousins Aurélie and Marcelline. One hot day I opened the refrigerator and was confronted by an ominous-looking pitcher of cloudy liquid, the refrigerator light refracted by its opaqueness. I asked my mother, "What is this?"

"It's sugar water," she replied. Perplexed, I asked her if someone forgot to finish making the lemonade. "No," she said in a hushed tone, "people here drink that for energy."

My tender age of six notwithstanding, surrounded by sugarcane fields, only one word came to mind, *slavery.* This empty calorie drink was probably older than lemonade itself, a necessity brought on by times I shuddered to imagine, much less accept. I was relieved to know that sugar water consumption was discontinued by our wing of the family when we moved north. Nevertheless, sugar as object and artifact, with a historical, symbolic, and interpretive power, has since persisted indelibly in my psyche.

While newly aware of this particular form of sugar consumption, I was still totally oblivious to the ways the global and the local shaped our own cultural forms of empty calorie consumption. While the pitcher of sugar water filled me with dread, I delighted in my Tantie's "German" chocolate cake, made with hand-shredded coconut fresh off the docks of New Orleans and enormous portions of delectable local pecans. We washed down our cake with cans of Hawaiian Punch. Before one cake was finished, another was baked. This was breakfast every day. At the end of that week, my mother and I had each gained seven pounds. I was in bayou Louisiana, the Tobacco Road of sugar, where nothing sweet could ever possibly be considered bad—despite the fact that cousins Aurélie, aged fourteen, and Marcelline, aged sixteen, weighed approximately 220 and 230 pounds, respectively.

How do I know? Because we discussed weight openly. It never occurred to us that being large would make one less desirable or less self-confident. Largeness was not seen as a barrier to life, marriage/partnership, children, family, or happiness. Weight gain, like sugar itself, was a ubiquitous condition of life, something that happened to you along the way. Sugar in the blood after breakfast and sugar water in the refrigerator for the rest of the day—that's our culture.

In fact, *sugar* was the term we used to refer to diabetes. But *sugar* also served as a term of warmth and affection, a personal pronoun, a verbal embrace that validates the sweetness of being one brings to life. It pays homage to the meaning it signifies within the family and wider community. The intimate social bonds experienced and labeled around sugar coexisted in relative cultural harmony with the fatalistic acceptance of "sugar" in the form of diabetes. But of course, it never occurred to my family, as with most of us, that we were subjects and citizens produced by histories, economies, and environments shaped by power.

This book shows that over time the racial categories created by the global sugar industry would soon come to be viewed as important data sites for learning more about Type 2 diabetes. Today, a multicolored multitude of corn syrup–sweetened "sugar water" beverages exist around the world, reflecting ever-penetrating corporate marketing influence with profound consequence, stressing public health efforts to address growing levels of obesity and Type 2 diabetes.[6] The connections between sugar production, labor, globalization, capital accumulation, and nutritional inputs and outcomes across divergent geographies—and the ways in which bodies, societies, and cultures are made and remade—echo strongly with my experiences as a member of a family embedded within these Creole histories, practices, racial categories, and relationships. Moreover, the story illustrates the complex social formations enabled by sugar, and hints toward sugar's making and remaking of both bodies and history.

STUDYING UP

My initial research intention aimed to examine the rise of Type 2 diabetes in a former Caribbean sugar-producing society. Preparatory archival and field research brought other, more necessary priorities to the fore. The more I researched Type 2 diabetes, the more acutely aware I became of both the technological and pharmaceutical interventions that were rapidly redefining the illness through the discourses they generated and circulated. I realized that I first needed to understand the clinical, market, and technological variables that were literally changing the face of Type 2 diabetes—as both a disease category and as a networking rubric around which subjects, markets, and practices are organized and recruited. Examining sugar as a racial project required an analytical shift from the sugar plantation to the boardrooms, research planning committees, and clinical spaces of the contemporary diabetes-industrial complex.[7]

To accomplish this, I decided upon a North American fieldwork project. In Laura Nader's words, my project became more "vertical" in its orientation and focus, enlisting medical anthropology and sociology, science and technology studies, and medical humanities perspectives in examining the institutional and market factors informing contemporary social understandings of Type 2 diabetes.[8] From 2008 to 2018, my multi-sited methodological approach involved five distinct sites. The first, the Diabetes Teaching Center at the University of California, San Francisco (UCSF), is considered one of the leading centers for diabetes education in the San Francisco Bay Area. I was interested in spending time with the center's staff looking at how they conducted diabetes education programs in a culturally and linguistically diverse area. I combined my embedded ethnography at UCSF during spring 2008 with comparative access to the Alameda County Department of Public Health.

This second component of the project began in summer 2008 and offered an opportunity to conduct participant observation and interviews among a comparatively larger African American population than San Francisco. In 2009, the Alameda County research led my inquiry from the technological confirmation of diagnosis, ex post facto, to the market-expanding possibilities of new Type 2 risk prediction technologies. This development led to the third part of the project, an examination of Tethys BioSciences, a biotechnology firm located in Alameda County. In late 2008, I learned from a public health professional about the company's efforts at recruiting an African American research cohort to test its new diabetes risk algorithm. Following this lead, I collected ethnographic, archival, and media analysis in Silicon Valley from 2009 to 2014. I wanted to better understand how the story of Tethys BioSciences mapped onto the historical emergence of venture capital financing, its relevance to biotechnology company funding, and provocative ways clinical data must both garner clinical approval and attract venture capital. I later discuss how and why value in this case lies not in the commodity but in the asset value of the company.

From 2009 to 2018, the fourth component of this project involved multi-sited public health and health disparities research in Chapel Hill, Houston, Baltimore, and Washington, DC. I combined participant observation, interviews, and archival research, as well as collaborative event ethnography (CEE) methodologically. CEE involved using diabetes events, health disparities conferences, and genomic research workshops as diverse field sites attracting a wide range of stakeholders.[9] This facilitated networking and subsequent interview opportunities with public health professionals, epidemiologists, molecular biologists, biological anthropologists, and geneticists of color working in diverse areas of health disparities research. The nine-year extended period of this research component reflects my reprioritization of the project after the precipitous fall in genomic sequencing costs in 2011 redefined notions of risk causation. It altered my research trajectory productively beyond race to argue for the analytical primacy of gender in considering the former. As I relate later, the 2013 mapping of the genome and epigenome of the HeLa mtDNA, originating from Henrietta Lacks, offered potential clues concerning the mechanisms by which maternal inherited mtDNA enabled metabolic adaptation to environmental change. The 2013 mapping refocused attention to the recurrent history of bioethical infringements upon black and female bodies. Against this bioethical backdrop, I frame the problem of recruiting sweetness emphatically as a problem embedded in sacrificial forms of racial and gendered exchange that re-create inequality.

The fifth research component, the upstate New York portion of my fieldwork, began in fall 2008 with yearly follow-up visits from 2009 to 2018. I chose the area because it had been a relatively prosperous region until the early 1980s, when local industries began laying off large numbers of workers—a process from which the area still seeks to recover. It is an area where the global realities of the contemporary economic situation have been slower to materialize. Behind this is a region ranked second in rates of hospitalizations and first in deaths due to liver cirrhosis and first in Type 2 death rates in the state, further exacerbated by an opioid epidemic that is taxing the local medical system beyond its limits.[10]

Diabetes is a complex, multifaceted illness that requires multisited engagement. I wanted to approach diabetes as a historical phenomenon where people, ideas, objects, technologies, capital, and institutional power have continually redefined and reshaped how the condition is experienced at the local (and the epidemiological) level. Instead of focusing primarily on communication within the health professional/patient relationship, I broadened my attention to consider how race, risk, and gender shape research recruitment strategies and the articulation of these concepts to families, communities, and populations by biotechnology, public health, and clinical institutions.

I also make the economic argument that race, Type 2 diabetes risk, and market risk are inextricably woven together. I suggest that high-risk Type 2 population groups unwittingly play an important role in adding value to both biotechnology and pharmaceutical commodities, which in turn are sold back to patients to manage their condition. I give equal attention to the relationship between the market and the forms of inclusive citizenship that recruitment demands, to consider the bioethical implications of these historical and continuing interactions between and intersections of race, ethnicity, class, and gender.

More boldly, *Sweetness in the Blood* challenges arguments claiming that collecting and filtering data according to racial categories offer the best approach to understanding, managing, and curing Type 2 diabetes. Over the last four centuries, social, political, and biological notions of race have accompanied an increasing global appetite for sugar. Enlightenment arguments about our common humanity also accompanied yet rendered hypocritical both sociopolitical and scientific musings about race, a critique written in blood.[11] The book fills a neglected ethnographic and historiographic gap between the sugar- and molasses-sweetened past of the enslaved African laborer and the high-fructose corn syrup and corporate-fed body of the contemporary consumer-laborer. In the following pages, I indict unequivocally assertions that notions of biological race constitute a conceptually relevant research driver of rational and legitimate scientific inquiry.

Therefore, studying Type 2 diabetes demands that I inhabit an ethnographic cross-section of biomedical, social scientific, and medical humanities fields simultaneously. This book weaves together all of these disciplinary approaches, along with African diaspora studies and black feminist scholarship in exploring how race, risk, and gender influence both social *and* technological definitions of diagnosis. This exploration involves an examination of how algorithms blur the interpretive lines between actionable diabetes risk and diagnosis in asymptomatic individuals. I link the phenomenon of diabetes risk technology with the emergence of genomic mapping technology and the gendered directionality the genomic turn makes toward sub-Saharan Africa. I employ these tools to highlight a temporal shift from diagnosis to individual risk, and from individual risk to ancestral risk. The following chapters show how African-descent groups found new relevance in Type 2 diabetes research, particularly as the identification and mapping of the wide genetic diversity of sub-Saharan populations has proceeded apace over the last quarter century. I highlight the ethical dilemmas researchers face in enrolling African-descent participation in health disparities research and their attempts at establishing trust and gaining consent, despite the historical realities of racial inequality, gendered dispossession, and scientific racism.

1

The At-Risk Ethnographer of Sweetness

We might continue this argument almost indefinitely going to one conclusion, that the Negro death rate and sickness are largely matters of condition and not due to racial traits and tendencies. . . .

—W. E. B. Du Bois, *Health and Physique of the Negro American*

In the summer of 2009, I met Darlene Pedraza[1] at a diabetes education class in Livermore, California. Her boss, Betty Washington, a diabetes educator working with the Alameda County Department of Public Health, had connected us. Over that summer, I was fortunate to shadow Darlene in the field, conduct interviews, and attend her classes. An energetic and knowledgeable teacher, Darlene and her associate, Hector Elizondo, offered to test me for Type 2 diabetes—at our first meeting. As an anthropologist, I found myself caught rather off-guard by the offer. Envisioning my initial involvement as more observation than participation, I was decentered from a presumably objective stance of analyzing to being analyzed. Subjectively, however, I began my project concerned about just how much the historical and genealogical legacies of sugar had manifested themselves biologically in my body. Membership in a high-risk group, academically induced corpulence, having had a diabetic grandmother and prediabetic mother, as well as the associated discourses of risk surrounding such pathological forms of racial kinship swirled through my mind. Deciding to face the "facts" with a mixture of curiosity and dread, I accepted the offer.

"This won't take but a minute, James," Hector said as I presented my arm. "Just think, only a few years ago you would have had to go to the clinic to take this test," he added. Using a portable hemoglobin A1C testing unit, field clinicians can now accurately measure the glucose metabolism of a red blood cell over the roughly three months of the cell's lifespan. This gives greater diagnostic reliability over other testing technologies. For example, a glucometer can only measure current blood-sugar levels, although newer models can store weeks' and months' worth of data, which can even be sent directly to the physician or clinician's office.

The finger prick was barely noticeable, hardly warranting mention. Having always been rather squeamish about needles and other invasive procedures, I was surprised at the relative absence of pain. Hector's assurance of a quick test was not taken as an assurance of a pain-free test. I had heard that line before and was prepared for the worst in terms of pain—and the worst in terms of diagnosis. So far, I was wrong about the needle. Now, for the result. Extracting not a vial but what I can only call a smidgen of blood, the HbA1c device took perhaps a minute to analyze my blood glucose metabolism. Or, at the very least, how it had been behaving metabolically over the course of the last three months. During that minute, I had uncontrollable visions of future performances of therapeutic contrition and penance: salads, bike rides, walking around Lake Merritt in Oakland every morning, yoga classes in Berkeley every evening, pilgrimages to farmers' markets every week, and a gym membership for everything in between. "5.1," Hector announced as the number flashed across the device screen, "Perfect!" Instantaneous joy and relief competed for my attention. However, an uncertain confusion punctuated these initial sentiments. Had I averted the pathologies of kinship? Were the vagaries of race and the specifics of relatedness lingering in the deeper biological recesses of my genetic and genomic destiny, waiting to emerge, waiting to strike?

In my case, a refusal to take the test carried its own risks against a larger backdrop of the stakes involved in conducting this research project. In terms of risk, refusal existed within a realm of predictive possibility that, due to my racial and familial histories, I could have missed the opportunity to definitively know about the state of my metabolic health. Yet regarding the stakes involved, my refusal could also have been seen as a personal protest against the predictive black box of racial determinism. Such a refusal would signal my rebellion against the racial categories that this book questions and seeks to make irrelevant regarding precisely which people develop Type 2 diabetes and how they develop the illness.

Much to Du Bois's certain chagrin, arguments linking racial traits and tendencies to disease have continued almost indefinitely. In the following pages, I interrogate race and risk as the primary, but flawed, technological drivers of Type 2 diabetes biomedical research recruitment. I explore the role of race in the development of diabetes technologies that move the epidemiological clock backward in time, from diagnosis to risk prediction of the asymptomatic individual. I take particular interest in how diagnostic and now predictive assessment technologies have served to rationalize new pharmaceutical interventions and regimes of blood glucose control.

Moving forward, I ask the reader to consider that the obesity and Type 2 diabetes pandemics arguably make moot any temptation to equate race with culture/nurture or biology/nature. Yet, scientific knowledge production based on recruitment outreach toward and data translated through racial categories has an antonymous, or contradictory, meaning. My primary argument in this book is that framing Type 2 diabetes risk as racially differentiated in terms of biology misses the conceptual mark: that Type 2 diabetes is a consequential physiological affect in relation to consumption and capital, reflecting new forms of behavior.

As both capitalized affect and phenomenology, inhabited racial risk, I argue, introduces the notion of a risk-managing subject.[2] The therapeutic epistemology driving this risk-managing subject, who is also a patient, consumer, and citizen, is the notion of choice, of agency. However, it is presumed that this laboring risk managing subject is a (bio)literate, rational actor whose choice and recruitment reflects the logic of risk aversion, or *care*, inherent to the choice itself.[3]

Sheila Jasanoff questioned the capability of economics, political science, and sociology to formulate a coherent language to describe the contemporary "co-production" of biotechnological development, social norms, and hierarchies.[4] The coproduction of science and society through recruitment and outreach requires a political-economic analysis to untangle the messiness of these collaborative and contested engagements. I do this by analyzing how a biotechnology company and a pharmaceutical clinical trial recruitment center each found public outreach to African-descent populations indispensable to their respective outreach projects. In both instances, attempts at successful outreach failed, leaving bare the cognitive dissonance and incommensurability resulting from a lack of social understanding about the African-descent populations they sought to engage.

A POLITICAL ECONOMY OF RACE AND RESEARCH

What I seek to show is that racial categories used in clinical, public health, and genetic/genomic research are as inherently unstable as earlier social scientific concepts of stable societies. I argue in this book, therefore, against notions of racial biologies. Race has no "essence," and in that important sense no "racial metabolism," to use sociologist Anthony Hatch's term, exists that can be expected to perform in a biologically distinct manner compared to other races in determining Type 2 risk.[5] Similarly, *Sweetness in the Blood* (re)defines "race" as a classificatory system of differentiated risks driven by political and economic forces that create new forms of biovalue.[6] In other words, race as a sociopolitical construct exists within larger political-economic structures of epidemiological consequence. I situate *Sweetness in the Blood* within a scholarly genealogy that began with Marx, Simmel, and Polanyi, up to the new economic moment cited by Jasanoff and expanded upon by later science and technology studies (S&TS) theorists engaging the intersections of political economy, biotechnological development, and scientific knowledge production.[7]

In using a political-economic approach, I engage the bundling of technology, ethnoracialization, and pharmaceuticalization in rationalizing market approaches to diabetes risk. My research foray into contemporary Type 2 diabetes required a disentangling of the different disciplinary and conceptual notions of risk driving different actors within and across social, economic, and scientific fields. These languages of risk inform each other with varying degrees of concordance. This does not mean that these languages of risk are either mutually intelligible or mutually aware.

In this section I begin the multidisciplinary untangling of risk, as articulated in anthropology, economics, and sociology, to describe the contemporary world we inhabit today and misinform sociotechnological linkages between race and risk. Douglas and Wildavsky's work on the dangers posed to and by those inhabiting various socially constructed spaces of risk, in its ethnographic data and analysis, has become a canonical text in the anthropology of risk.[8] They remind us that all effective healing involves ritual within a space where disorder, impurity, discord, and the socially constructed perceptions of the dangers or risks they represent can be rectified. In his classic on economic risk, Franklin Knight[9] argued that economic risk in relation to profit can be defined as "measurable uncertainty," or, better still, "true uncertainty." What is interesting about Knight's notion of economic risk as grounded in quantitative assessment is that he relegated *qualitative* risk to the realm of immeasurable uncertainty. Immeasurable uncertainty, he argued, must be analytically distinguished from *true* uncertainty, or risk. Of note, Knight saw his work firmly grounded in economics as a social science, a study in method, of how social organization could better drive economic cooperation in the pursuit of improving social life.

In this pursuit, Knight argued for bracketing out either a defense or a critique of the capitalist system. It was his opinion that without first completely understanding the system under examination, capitalism should be neither prematurely valorized nor devalued. Yet, within Knight's conceptual and methodological parameters, left outstanding was an examination of power, control, and affect, both economic and social. Needless to say, a political economic critique of the epidemiological consequences of power and affect remained unexplored.

Later, Ulrich Beck extended Knight in arguing for a necessary distinction between economic and sociological notions of risk.[10] Beck placed emphasis on the question of power and control. He argued that regimes of control based upon calculable forms of predictive risk should be differentiated from incalculable forms of risk without precedent. The rationality of the former cannot anticipate the irrationality of the latter. Both forms of risk, the calculable and the incalculable, Beck maintained, comprise the contemporary risk-saturated world we inhabit. Inhabiting risk, therefore, is a means of both being and being ruled in the contemporary world.[11]

W. E. B. Du Bois argued that race and self-identification inhere themselves to a political economy of productive instability within fields of power. Simply stated, for Du Bois, the shifting winds of political and economic fortune reshape individual, social, and scientific notions of race.[12] Nevertheless, technological innovation continues alongside persistent narratives linking illness risk with notions of race.[13] Over the last two decades, technological innovations and resurgent discussions about race and risk have occurred during a robust period of pharmaceutical company expansion.[14] Some scholars have noted the ways race and risk intersect with biomedical practice and pharmaceutical development rationales.[15] Despite the fact that all humans share 99.93 percent genetic affinity, genetic and genomic research continues to focus on the 0.07 percent genetic difference among human populations. This epistemological stance furthers both discursive and methodological scientific practices driving medical research through the biological prisms of race and sex. These stances inform patient epistemology concerning health access and health disparities in terms of the subjective experience of patienthood, and the objective reality of epidemiological data.[16]

Drawing on Weber's "irrationality of rationalization," Duana Fullwiley argues that biomedical research based on race "runs the risk of irrationalizing both" (emphasis removed) medicine and race.[17] As Du Bois understood in 1940, the instability of racial categories lays bare the irrationality of sociocultural preconceptions about human difference as open to biological explanation. Du Bois's political economy of sociobiological race, and the dialectical relationship between racial classification and (self-)identification, echoed into early-twenty-first-century health disparities scholarship. This new "inclusion-and-difference" paradigm is driven by older epistemes of intergroup variation as biologically ascertainable in terms of "race"; this is evidenced by the paucity of research extrapolating genetic research across heterogeneous populations and ethnoracial categories. Challenging the notion of biological race, anthropologist Michael Montoya interrogated the ways in which genetic researchers allocate clinical meaning to DNA fragments assigned to poorly defined ethnic and racial populations. Of importance, Montoya argues that ethnographers need to attend to racial categorization as a research method to better understand how genetics researchers imbue biological attributes with racialized meaning.[18]

As I will relate in subsequent chapters, the original Framingham Study's white research subjects have new phenotypical company with which they now share political and biomedical research space.[19] However, previous epistemological and methodological errors remain intact: "race" as a genotypically fixed final destination (or stable category, in equilibrium) that is scientifically discoverable, rather than the moving target that it really is. In this way, race operates as an irrational yet intractable *method* in social and scientific categorization that generates economic value already embedded historically within longer-standing cultural modes of exchange. As such, racialized approaches to generating scientific production appear rational, leaving critics of these methods open to accusations that they are questioning science itself.[20]

Within science and technology studies, some scholars have expressed new terms to describe the ways capital has been reconfigured along novel lines of biological valuation based on new modes of exchange.[21] Kaushik Sunder Rajan notes the emergence of *biocapital,* a confluence of the life sciences, venture capital, and technology. Commercial capital and venture capital produce different knowledge demands and products, but both reproduce structures of capitalisms, writ plural, reflecting different modes of capitalistic production. Contestation and cooperation over what constitutes public and private knowledge drive the creative tension behind the generation of biocapital.[22] I draw on Sunder Rajan, while I am also mindful of Birch and Tyfield's important critique of what they call "bioconcepts" as overdetermined by S&TS theorists. They argue that misplaced analytical attention on technoscientific and biological objects elide a necessary engagement with the political economy of recent changes in the financial system undergirding what the authors prefer to call "the bioeconomy."[23]

I argue here that race, coproduced by constructed social norms and hierarchies of risk and value, must factor into analyses of the scientific amalgam of society, technology, and economics. However, Sunder Rajan made a specific argument: an analysis of the political economy of exchange, or for that matter the item of exchange, carries epistemic, discursive, and, in the case of biocapital, institutional notions of value.[24] These notions of value are consequential of structural articulations and idiomatic forms (or categories) of *grammar.*[25] Morrison and Cornips use the term "promissory futures" to describe these speculative language strategies, which biotechnology companies deploy to attract venture capital funding. As we shall explore in later chapters, speculative language futures are both tentative and problematic, a condition of inhabiting the risk worlds of contemporary political, economic, and technosocial life.[26]

Both Knight and Beck pointed to the technologies of risk that make possible advancements in the risk assessment methodologies and interpretive schematics to which they both alluded. They both accurately pointed to the productive, even profitable, ambiguities generated through risk assessment, which the postevent (or for our purposes, diagnosis) could not achieve in the past. Despite Knight's insistence on risk research as part of an overall improvement in social life, his argument failed to take into account the disruptive social consequences that economic rationales of risk and profit can wreak upon societies, markets, and bodies. Later, Beck normalized this disruptive capability as a rationalized principle of power, society, and the body.[27] However, both Knight and Beck elided a critical discussion about the ways social scientific estimations of risk, power, and social facts intersect with longer histories and culturally embedded moral economies of racialized and gendered forms of exchange and participation.

Sweetness in the Blood details the ways diabetes research recruitment reveals the ongoing reification of racial categories that highlight unequal socioeconomic relationships of unequal value. Further, it offers a lens for examining how diabetes risk gets read as racial risk—in other words, how culture as practices misinform historical attributions of black pathology as inherently biological and perennially valuable.

THE RACIAL BIOLOGY OF THE BLACK ATLANTIC

Sidney Mintz identified the origins of the Industrial Revolution in sugarcane production. He linked this to consumption in Europe, specifically Britain, and to capital, which made possible the triangular trade in slaves, sugar, and textiles. For Mintz, the Caribbean is an emergent site of protoindustrialism and the creation of new subjectivities of production and consumption under exploitative capital. The first time an English factory worker drank sweetened tea was a significant historical event of symbolic, economic, and social transformative power, and for the purposes of this book, metabolic consequence.

In the Introduction, I purposely included Louisiana within this geo-theoretical rubric. I do this both to contextualize my theoretical application of creolization and to critique the absence of any sustained scholarly engagement to deterritorialize and denationalize disciplinary discourses rooted in U.S. black exceptionalism. I take this tack not only to highlight both the historical fluidity of black migration in the circum-Atlantic and the geographic range of the global sugar industry, but also, as I show in later chapters, to reflect the increasing diversity of the black population and its scientific relevance in the contemporary United States. In this way, I use the term *African American* in a hemispheric, not a nationalistic sense. I do this for three important reasons: (1) to trouble bounded biocultural narratives of U.S. blackness, (2) to illustrate the morphological dynamism of an inherently unstable racial category, and (3) to highlight the challenges that narratives of bounded racial categories present in terms of achieving cultural competence (CC), effectively communicating biomedical knowledge to the public, and re-creating the epistemological and methodological errors of assumed racial biologies.

I direct this quest by posing several questions: What is race? What is risk? How does history inform both and intersect with contemporary notions of Type 2 diabetes risk as racially differentiated? I begin with an exploration of how sugar serves as both a metaphor for diabetes and a theoretical generator of anthropological notions of difference. As a cultural anthropologist, I endeavor in this book to examine the ways the social life of sugar as a material product has changed nutritional destinies and shaped metabolic futures across the globe.[28] But as a medical anthropologist, I also wish to explicate sugar as an illness metaphor for diabetes, what I call *pathological sweetness*. Hence, I situate sugar as both material and metaphor theoretically within a larger narrative of race.

In this task, I have broadened my theoretical reach to include scholarship on the Caribbean, as well as diasporic and transnational perspectives to better grapple with the diverse forms of global metabolic modernity that have emerged from within Creole societies over the last five hundred years.[29] For example, Indian Ocean sugar-plantocracies also used enslaved West African labor and were in geographic proximity to the historical sites of original sugarcane cultivation and consumption in South and Southeast Asia. Further, linguistic research sources the development of the Afro-French Creole language (spoken formerly) in Louisiana, and today in Réunion, to a common origin in Senegal in the eighteenth century.[30] In later chapters I discuss how Indian Ocean Afro-Creole bodies were seen as indispensable barometers for measuring Type 2 diabetes risk in a genetically diverse population.

Anthropology's historical disinterest in the Caribbean, a region marked by "nothing but contact," was a methodological problematic of globalization that obscured the discipline's preoccupative search for culturally isolated and easily essentialized groupings of people, bounded linguistically, geographically, historically, and epistemologically.[31] The Caribbean's unique global and transnational connective circuitries made it unsuitable ethnographic and theoretical territory, as it contained "all the wrong people from all the wrong places."[32] Sidney Mintz located this disciplinary act of misrecognition in North American racial discourses and early twentieth-century politics: North

American anthropologists of the time occupied a habitus of racial and spatial social exclusivity that "made their black fellow citizens alien without making them exotic."[33]

DIASPORA, RACE, AND THE TRANSNATIONAL BODY

In contesting racialized risk, I write in this book against notions of African "retentions" as articulated by anthropologist Melville Herskovits, who argued that a psychosomatic cultural unity exists among and between African-descent groups in the African diaspora. Herskovits was engaged in the noble project of refuting Hegel by bringing Africa into history. However, while his project sought to privilege culture over race, he inadvertently rebiologized both through a search for an essential Africa within black bodies.[34] I seek to avoid any implicit phenotypical conflation of cultural "retentions" as somehow biological or, for that matter, behavioral. While sympathetic to Herskovits's attempt at demonstrating a persistent and significant African sociohistorical presence, I am careful in this book not to equate biology with either culture or race.

Entrenched attitudes on both sides of the racial frontlines make such an argument difficult to promote. As Martinican author Edouard Glissant wrote in the case of Louisiana, "Whites from Louisiana generally refuse to admit any such connections . . . between the linguistic, material, structural, and African elements they share, not only with blacks in the area, but in the Caribbean as well." In his experience, "you cite a whole list for a skeptical audience that does not wish to know that its history travels with the seas."[35]

Nevertheless, sugar production, consumption, and subsequent metabolic affect disturb and disabuse ahistorical notions of racial insularity from physiological change and diabetes risk. Therefore, as a project in cultural, not racial, geography, I take seriously Paul Gilroy's earlier assertion of the need for a broader-based scholarship throughout the diasporic culture area he called the Black Atlantic. Nationalist, ethnic, and linguistic particularities should not, in Gilroy's estimation, obscure the commonalities of history, practice, and their newer, globalized cultural phenomena in the postmodern black present. In other words, history, practice, and the present transcend reductionist phenotypical attributions.[36] Therefore, in arguing against racialized diabetes risk, I also argue against race.[37]

James Clifford, in dialogue with Gilroy and echoing Glissant, "insists on the routing of diaspora discourses in specific maps/histories. Diasporic subjects are distinct versions of modern, transnational, and intercultural experience. Thus historicized, diaspora cannot become a master trope or 'figure' for modern, complex, or positional identities, cross-cut and displaced by race, sex, gender, class, and culture."[38] "Tradition," "the nation," and "difference" can also be seen as historically (re)constructed by social actors within fields of power across political economies of time and space.[39] The displacement of groups across time and space reinvents categories as well as the groups themselves. Power reinvents history and fragments memories both imagined and recovered piecemeal through acts of identification (i.e., *slave-descendent, African American, Jamaican*) rather than identity (i.e., *Yoruba*), and through relationships (i.e., *black*) rather than as essentialized forms (i.e., *African*).[40]

Understanding sugar historically and consequentially as a global enterprise in human metabolic engineering requires diasporic and transnational understandings of change and affect to unbind nationalist narratives of race, risk, and scientific knowledge production. In this respect, I write mindfully and carefully about the term *diaspora,* what Jacqueline Nassy Brown called "the most abused term in the study of black folks here and there."[41] This book offers a medical anthropology approach to trouble scholarship situated within a corpus of fragmented memories (Caribbean anthropology and nationalist history, diaspora, transnational and cultural studies, postmodern and postcolonial studies) characterized by searches for cultural origins, racial identity, slave society, resistance, and so on in ways that, in agreement with Trouillot, privilege a move toward cultural studies and away from ethnography. This can become a never-ending search, risking further essentialization of both the past and those putative groups categorically and analytically ossified within that past. In this respect, Herskovits's project is still very much alive, often without the benefit of fieldwork, as racial and cultural theories tenaciously remain the two paths most taken in analyzing both society and biology.[42]

(BIO)CREOLIZATION AND ITS DISCONTENTS

Jacqueline Nassy Brown calls attention to the ways "diaspora" serves as a totalizing catchment of uncritical inclusion that in effect serves to negate and police its collapsed definitional boundaries without due regard to context, particularity, and nuance.[43] Interdisciplinary work on *creolization* and *African retentions* sheds light on how each term has come to insinuate diaspora as biological exception instead of affirming cultural diversity as the general state of nature. This problematizes efforts to delink race from risk as it reinforces racial categorization, the biopolitics of the nation-state, and the bioeconomy of the global venture capital market.

Much of the scholarship on creolization in diaspora studies has tended to reproduce the bounded racial essentialisms that anthropologists Sidney Mintz and Richard Price warned against. For example, Viranjani Munasinghe argued correctly that creolization as a sociohistorical process traditionally examined Caribbean societies through a dual European/African lens that left little analytical room for East Indians. Earlier Marxist-inspired preoccupations with dialectical oppositions based on European/African, master/slave dyads were too neatly convenient and exclusionary. The same theorists and ethnographers who argued for a historical approach to understanding social diversity failed to extend this methodology beyond a reified, Afro-European analytic continuum. Munasinghe saw Mintz and Price's definition of creolization, based on plantation interactions between Europeans and Africans, as overdetermined, in that it left little room to theorize Indian (and for that matter Chinese and Lebano-Syrian) life in the Caribbean as part of larger, ongoing processes of creolization that have occurred postslavery.[44]

Other scholars in Caribbean and diaspora studies have taken up the question of creolization in heterogeneous societies. Aisha Khan prefers the notion of "mixing" to creolization; in contrast, Shalini Puri's deconstruction of the social politics of creolization uses the term "hybridity."[45] For Puri, hybridity exists in two forms: cultural and racial. Noting that cultural hybridity is a social fact in Trinidad, Puri locates racial "hybridity" in the person of the *Dougla*, the offspring of Afro- and Indo-Trinidadian parents.[46] However, in this analysis cultural diversity as a biosocial fact is elided in favor of a definition of hybridity as a novel categorical exception rooted in a bounded notion of racial biology that presumes racial purity. In short, as an item of social analysis, cultural diversity as a social fact was not seen as the de-facto regenerator of biological diversity as the general state of nature.

In the Caribbean, immigrant Indian populations from various parts of North, East, and South India have collapsed into a generic "Indian" biopolitical category. Even Munasinghe admittedly was not immune from diasporic inclusion through labeling while in the field: Despite her Sri Lankan Buddhist background and repeated efforts at clarification, both Indo-and Afro-Trinidadians read her as "Indian."[47] Like enslaved Africans in the New World who came to embody a cross-section of African groups spanning vast distances of West and Central Africa, so have most of the Indian subcontinental population, notably in Trinidad, Guyana, and Surinam. Biomedical, cultural, and social scientific disciplines in Trinidad tend to use this umbrella category "Indian" unreflexively. As in relation to enslaved Africans, creolization as a theory of labor in relation to capital strikes similarly here, with both groups "exchanging their country marks" for the reified biopolitical ethnoracial label and its attendant socioeconomic concerns.[48]

Therefore, in addressing the theoretical privileging of static racial biologies over dynamic cultural practices, anthropologist Bill Maurer, echoing Marilyn Strathern, is wary:

> My main concern with the adoption of creolization discourse is that when it takes on the hybridity rubric and not the grammatical formulation of Mintz and Price (for example), it tends to replicate an idiom of relatedness, relationship, and the idea of relation itself (intellectual, genealogical, and so on), tightly bound with the biogenetic model of Euro-American kinship, and thus naturalizes itself.[49]

My insistence in this book on a nonbiological equivocation of creolization, diaspora, race, and admixture echoes Maurer's discomfort with notions like *the Black Atlantic, hybridity, mixing, mestizaje,* and so on, in that they reproduce the biogenetic essentialisms and associated linguistic metaphors definitive of Herskovitsian anthropology and scientific racism.[50] In short, they create and proliferate increasingly microscopic forms of *othering* that fascinate both social and biological scientists alike. We will later examine how the idea of racial *admixture* has been further strengthened by new genetic and postgenomic technologies that highlight the intractability of concepts linking race and biology used in diabetes research, testing, and therapeutics.[51]

I understand that by using Mintz and Price's definition of creolization as a cultural theory of labor in relation to capital, and not a scientific theory of racial biology, I take up the task of persuasively delinking race from risk. I direct this task to the examination of Type 2 diabetes to argue for the universality of diabetes risk. In making that argument, I join Glissant and Gilroy in centering *blackness, diaspora,* and *creolization* not upon phenotype but the ethno-, techno-, and market-scapes within which culture is mutually produced, consumed, and embodied through circuits of travel, media, migration, and exchange. In critiquing the research recruitment gaze on black bodies, I situate both Type 2 diabetes and diaspora within overlapping geographies of practice, not bounded biologies of race.

I make the argument that diabetes risk should not be defined by genetics or race, as science continues to show. But that hasn't impacted how the diabetes industry is or has been reaching out to potential research participants/consumers. Why?—Because of the market value of certain target populations. *Sweetness in the Blood* chronicles how outreach by both scientific and industry actors to African-descent populations skews knowledge production about the illness, instead of following an approach that seeks to understand Type 2 diabetes as a global phenomenon, one in which African-descent populations form part of an evaluative continuum of statistical means, modes, averages, and outliers of risk independent of ethnic and racial classification.

TRANSLATING THE WRONG BODY INCORRECTLY

Anthropological scholarship on translation has examined the social production of incommensurability, or the inability to bridge gaps in understanding between two or more sets of actors. Briggs and Hallin suggest that new categories of risk are created through forms of inclusive citizenship based on notions of biologized difference.[52] Built upon their earlier discursive model, or authoritative proficiency in targeting audiences based on difference and communicating risk to these audiences through the lens of difference, Briggs and Hallin point to a dual process of racialization and medicalization.[53] Incommensurability is built into Briggs and Hallin's model, in which both translational medicine and public health outreach are poorly communicated to and misunderstood by individual patients in private spaces and to the public in public spaces. In short, efforts achieving cultural competence in medical communication occur on the social field of combat. As an ideology of power, incommensurability circulates, not only to targeted audiences, but also through and among these audiences, then back to their discursive progenitors. Locating expertise and claims to narrative authority amid the social hubris of dissonance and incommensurability troubles the discursive circulation of medical risk based on difference. Communicating science not only reconfigures nature but who is situated where and how securely within its confines.

Elizabeth Povinelli argued:

> Through different symbolic forms of communication, people receive various messages as to how they should calculate and calibrate the stakes, pleasures, and risks of being a certain type of form in a certain type of formed space. Drawn into the semiotic process are the formal and inform(ation)al institutional forces that dictate the varying degrees of pleasure and harm varying types of people face breaking frame—of having the wrong body, or wrong form of a body, or wrong attitude about that formed body in a (informed) formed world.[54]

Creolization and admixture, biohistorical products of "all the wrong people from all the wrong places," tell a story of just who has the "wrong body" in terms of diabetes risk. It appears that African descendants, Indigenous, Latino, and Asian/Pacific Islander populations, in comparison to white Europeans, all possess the wrong body to inherit, but the right body for clinical research, diabetes education, and public health stakeholders. The main threads of this story will show that historical forms of racial and gendered exchange regarding black bodies, both under the biomedical gaze and patriarchal capital surveillance, continue to operate based upon novel imaginaries of difference based on sub-Saharan ancestry. We will explore how genetic and genomic research complicate this story about an illness that carries no inherent racial risk, yet which, due to the genetic diversity of sub-Saharan populations, offers a geometrically larger pool of diverse DNA to study in the search to discover the possible genetic mechanisms driving Type 2 diabetes causation. In this effort, we will need to trouble older phenotypical notions of blackness, Africa, and sub-Saharan genetic inheritance to resituate the biological and the geographical attributions of these terms to show that they, as with creolization, have been found outside of, and arguably exist as well as Africa within admixed bodies.

In particular, the cellular dynamism of one admixed/Creole maternal African descendent, Henrietta Lacks, portends to provide a clearer lens toward understanding the evolutionary metabolic adaptations of humanity to diverse environments. Her story highlights the unequal forms of exchange and wealth production buttressed by social and historical forms of labor and hierarchical claims to expertise. Our analytical journey interrogates whether the biological and social relationships and histories of exchange characterizing creolization evidence Type 2 diabetes as a cultural theory of labor in relation to capital, or a scientific theory of racial biology.

RACE, GENDER, AND THE MATRIARCHAL GIFT

Classical anthropology defined gift exchange as a circulation of property that sets in motion obligations to give, receive, and reciprocate.[55] Early functionalist projects focused on exchange through a social and political lens from which the value of the gift was seen as secondary to the function it served in cementing human relationships. However, women and slaves have each been exchanged historically as both transferable gifts and property.[56] W. E. B. Du Bois's theorization of the gift as racial labor preceded Marcel Mauss's better known notion of the gift as political.[57] I read Du Bois's definition of the gift alongside Catherine Waldby's account of twenty-first-century "tissue economies," in which cells and tissues are transferred from poor, socially and economically disadvantaged "surplus" bodies to the wealthy and powerful in society, a transfer rationalized by narratives of citizenship and civic duty.[58] And like Du Bois, Waldby puts forward a redistributive and regenerative political economy for bodies made deficient in their material appropriation. Participatory inclusion by the poor and disadvantaged, particularly women, highlights Joan Scott's insistence upon placing gender front and center in any historical analysis of labor.[59] Additionally, I bring the notion of racialized forms of gendered labor as negotiable property, to bear on Richard Hyland's assertion that gift giving and exchange occur in sociocultural spaces outside and in spite of legal or moral sanction, where, according to Karla Holloway, "the evolution of legal text did not . . . fully and /or finally determine social act."[60]

Outside of critical race and feminist studies and the medical humanities, few scholars have engaged the ways notions of matriarchy both inform conditions of exchange and misrecognize affective kinship structures. The story of Henrietta Lacks and its embeddedness in slavery's historical rupturing of personhood generally, and self-agency specifically, troubles neat scholarly notions of gift exchange, reciprocation, and consent, by introducing a body that has historically constituted a "point of convergence where biological, sexual, social, cultural, linguistic, ritualistic, and psychological fortunes join."[61] Racial and gender constructs overdetermine notions of individual sovereignty and subjectivity for women and blacks, whose bodies always have had "a compromised relationship to privacy."[62]

Genomic science offers new opportunities to make private bodies public, often under the neoliberal banner of individual sovereignty. Sometimes this sovereignty is defined in terms of an "inclusion-and-difference" paradigm, which is driven by older epistemes circumscribing group difference in terms of biologically ascertainable "races."[63] However, "race" is still often rendered a genotypically fixed feature of the body (or a stable category, in equilibrium) that is scientifically discoverable, rather than an elusive or illusive target. This presents an intractable form of social and scientific classification that Alondra Nelson suggests has created new forms of social meaning around identity: Genetic tests as a commodity offer new tools for "self-fashioning" based on notions of scientific impartiality and fulfilling one's "genealogical aspirations."[64] While Nelson cautions against prematurely assessing the social and political ramifications of newly marketed genetic "ancestry" testing models, she submits that the knowledge claims they make, as well as their subsequent interpretation by consumers, set in motion new forms of subjectification and self-recruitment based on biological notions of racial difference.[65]

The personal fulfillment of diasporic genealogical aspirations and the political imperatives of research inclusion underline a desire to make legible ancestries violently ruptured by slavery and colonialism and bodies marked anonymous historically. In particular, black feminist writers, specifically fiction writers, make visible these otherwise violent and anonymous historical silences and ellipses of memory. In Toni Morrison's *Beloved,* the novel's protagonist, Sethe, attempts unsuccessfully to repress traumatic memories of slavery, bondage, and loss, which involved murdering her own two-year-old daughter to prevent her recapture by slave patrols pursuing runaway slaves in the north.[66]

Saidiya Hartman writes about the tension between slavery, memory, and the archive, and how each produces both contingent silences and a sense of irrevocable ancestral loss. She asks, "Was my hunger for the past so great that I was now encountering ghosts? Had my need for an entrance into history played tricks on me, mocked my scholarly diligence, and exposed me as a girl blinded by mother loss?"[67] In writing about the violent erasure of genealogical memory, Hartman blurs fiction with historical analysis—what elsewhere she calls "critical fabulation"[68]—to excavate an unknowable maternal past. The erasures of memory and history instituted by racial slavery continued to haunt the mortal life of Henrietta Lacks and the immortal life of the HeLa cells taken from her, both situated in "a common historical ground, the socio-political order of the New World" in which, according to Hortense Spillers, a "diasporic plight marked a theft of the body."[69] The Lacks narrative represents the private theft of the mortal black body that can be "killed," while HeLa represents an "immortal" public text read from genetic analyses of the cells, their genome, and their epigenome, all decoded from, to paraphrase Spillers, "an undecipherable kind of hieroglyphics of Black flesh."[70]

This book takes up the task of bringing together the very different but mutually dependent bioeconomic and sociopolitical attempts to decipher black bodies in the effort to learn more about Type 2 diabetes. We will see that as technological advances make new claims about both race and Type 2 risk, the hieroglyphics of black flesh have become more difficult to decode, as both the biological location of race and risk continue to elude researchers. The social dynamics of the racial category also continue to defy definition, due to immigration, internal migration, and ever-deepening kinship ties between and among racial groups within the "one-drop" rule of U.S. history.

So, I present a paradox to the reader: How to reconcile the current sociomedical milieu that presumes racial risk for a nonselective illness of global epidemic proportions, Type 2 diabetes, with the fact that one particular "race" embodies global genetic diversity itself? At the core of our conversation is the question of ethical research inclusion given centuries of unrequited black and female labor. The book expands then to transcend older debates about inclusion to center a response based on the possibility of justice as an insistent socioeconomic prerequisite criterion to entreaties to enroll, participate, and exchange in the face of entrenched social forms of unequal and sacrificial exchange. What does the relative absence of justice—social, economic, and medical—mean within the context of inclusion? And of contemporary importance, how does the increased diversity of researchers complexify notions of medical justice and research inclusion?

THE JOURNEY

I offer this book as an intellectual invitation to think through the assumptions behind the clinical and biotechnology recruitment of African American and African-descent populations for Type 2 diabetes research. It is not a metanarrative of the phenomenon, but rather a composite ethnographic picture of contemporary biotechnology and clinical research framings of Type 2 diabetes risk and race. Chapter 2 gives a historical and genealogical overview of how diabetes has been researched, understood, and framed racially over the last century. Specifically, I focus on diabetes's classificatory history and the technological advances that have moved people, technologies, and markets from clinical diagnostic confirmation to clinical risk-predictive calculation.

Chapter 3 chronicles one company's efforts to recruit U.S. African Americans to test their new diabetes risk-score algorithm in hopes of increasing the clinical and market value of their technology. I show how extant racial categories and their scientifically imagined members were seen as important research populations of risk to both biotechnology and biomedical researchers. I present an ethnographic narrative of the ethical and translational challenges affecting this company's recruiting efforts. I argue that while neoliberal discourses of diversity and inclusion have increased the biovalue of these populations, in this case African Americans, a translational wall of distrust still exists between research communities and targeted risk groups.[71]

Chapter 4 explores the historical and contemporary factors affecting African American apprehension and reticence toward participating in biomedical research and the problematic role churches play as a recruitment venue. I show how the Tuskegee Syphilis Study resonates in the social body of the community, and the contingent role that African American churches play in communicating the biomedical message. Of equal importance, I argue that professional representations of biomedical messages within a church venue allow, problematically, for greater acceptance of public health Type 2 discourses and programs toward limited demographic groupings. I suggest that the African American church, while not monolithic, remains the institutional center of real and imagined African American life.[72]

Chapter 5 examines race and health disparities in light of recent advances in genomic sequencing technology and the rationale undergirding the growing significance of African-descent populations in genomic sampling recruitment. I show that race served as a proxy in population narratives of diversity, sub-Saharan ancestry, and admixture. I submit that historical inequalities embedded within these narratives reflect complex sets of social relationships of biological consequence. These social relationships, I will summarize, shape forms of exchange and notions of trust. I conclude in emphasizing that genomic research into sub-Saharan ancestry and admixture underlines the primary importance of analyzing gender before attempting to understand the notion of race. No other disease reveals this importance more than Type 2 diabetes.

CATEGORICAL INCLUSION: SCRIPTING INEQUALITY

Michael Montoya frames the term *bioethnic conscription* in seeking to define the ways the clinical research gaze viewed biological heritability through socially constructed racial categories:

> Rather, bioethnic conscription is a practice with at least two modes, one descriptive and the other attributive. In the first mode, ethnic and racial, hereafter referred to as ethnoracial classifications, are used to pragmatically describe human groups. They are used, for instance, to report to readers of scientific publications from which human groups the biological samples and data sets were derived for the study. The naming of human groups is a matter of method. In the latter mode, ethnoracial labels do more than identify groups: The labels are used to attribute qualities to groups. Attribution modifies, often in a delimiting way, what it refers to.[73]

Although *attribution* and *ascription* approach synonymy, particularly regarding Montoya's description of scientific epistemology and practice, attribution does not fully convey the breadth of the total social field foregrounding such attitudes and practices. Further, as Montoya correctly argues, "Attribution modifies, often in a delimiting way, what it refers to." However, I suggest that *attribution* delimits social inequalities embedded within biological samples and data sets used in research. I use the social scientific term *ascription* rather than *attribution* to analytically engage the wider hierarchal social system of inequality informing research gleanings of both the biological sample and the data set. While embracing the notion of "bioethnic conscription" as a *descriptive* form of scientific ethnoracial classification and attribution, I seek to expand my analytical inquiry to the wider social field. In the remainder of this book, I aim to link estimations of racialized risk with inherited status as an *explanatory* form of ascriptive inequality marking not only ethnorace, but also kinship, gender, and class.

The scriptural and moral authority to account for and validate difference, once the province of theology and philosophy, later claimed in the nineteenth century by biology, ethnology, and anthropology, today exists in biogenetic articulations of human variation.[74] As with the creolization rubric mentioned earlier, what has not changed is the notion of human diversity as molecularized states of exception rather than the general state of nature. These molecular states of exception persist in the form of racial categories utilized as explanatory models of both disease risk and disease incidence.[75] Categorical racial thinking also serves to operationalize research and intervention strategies. While race as an imprecise theory remains prominent, I direct ultimate attention to how racial recruitment has become an imprecise method for achieving measurable research, market, and public health outcomes. The notion of a "racial metabolism," this book argues, exemplifies the ways race as theory and racial recruitment as practice occlude a broader understanding of Type 2 diabetes as an illness that arises from an array of social, environmental, and economic factors.[76] I emphasize that although I reject notions of an inherent racial metabolism, a refusal I link dually with that of Herskovits's African retentions, I will show that sub-Saharan African ancestry offers new ways of ascribing both risk and value to the diabetes research enterprise.[77]

I conclude, doubtful that developing trust in an increasingly diverse African American research population can occur in a sociopolitical milieu that reproduces the static racial category itself. Such an attempt superimposes medical equality superficially upon recalcitrant social attitudes and practices of racial stigmatization. Further, I suggest that bioscientific deployment of racial categories in translational research rationalizes social and cultural notions of racial difference as scientifically valid. The approach to Type 2 diabetes highlights the persistence of categorical thinking about race and risk in public health, clinical, and biotechnological research.

Note that I would have preferred to italicize African American(s) in this book to contest biological assertions of race as well as to highlight the political, economic, and spatial factors that have historically shaped the category. By inclusion, I would also have italicized Latino, white/Caucasian, Native American, and so on in attempting to refocus critical attention to the effects of power and its invisible capacity to author visible narratives of biological and phenotypical ascription. However, in this process of italicized ascription, I would have scarcely conveyed both my own ambiguity and duplicity in the matter. Ambiguity, in that as an anthropologist, I do not subscribe to theories of biological race. This theoretical refusal is embedded within the critique I seek to make in this book concerning the ways in which race is envisioned and translated epidemiologically in clinical research, biotechnology, and public health arenas. On the other hand, by scripturally referencing racial categories, I admit duplicity by participating in both their historic and contemporary reproduction. I aim to trouble this conformed duplicity with a critical ambiguity that productively highlights the instability of constructed racial categories and the partial understandings these knowledge claims allow and restrict from their conceptually unstable data silos.

2
Sweet Blood
INVENTING THE PREDIABETIC

> In recent years there have been numerous surmises
> concerning the nature of the genetic readjustments man
> must make to his rapidly changing environment. Genes
> and combinations of genes which were at one time an
> asset may in the face of environmental change become
> a liability.
> —James Neel, "Diabetes Mellitus: A 'Thrifty' Genotype
> Rendered Detrimental by 'Progress'?"

Studying "sugar" or diabetes and the physiological effects of pathological sweetness on the human body has occupied the attention of
medical practitioners throughout recorded history. Diabetes as an illness has been recognized for over four millennia in various medical
systems and cultures, from ancient Egypt to classical India, China,
Greece, and Rome. Known in Sanskrit as *Madhumedha,* it shares the
same descriptive diagnostic nomenclature as its Latin counterpart,
diabetes mellitus: sweet urine. More precisely, both *madhu* and *mel*
mean *honey* in their respective languages. It should be noted that by
the third century BCE, classical Ayurvedic medicine in India recognized over twenty different types of diabetes.[1] Traditional medical
systems located diabetic pathology diagnostically in the kidneys and
directed therapeutic attention to that organ.

In the West, the kidney also remained the organ of evaluative attention well into the twentieth century. Clinically, the diagnosis and
monitoring of diabetes was performed through urinalysis until the
late 1970s. This method of biological assessment was conducted to
monitor hyperglycemia (high blood glucose) and address diabetes
symptoms and complications: polyuria (excessive urination), noctu-
ria (excessive night-time urination), and polydipsia (excessive thirst).

At this point in time in the 1970s, glycemic control was not a therapeutic goal—clinically or pharmaceutically.

The discovery of insulin in 1923 and its physiological role in glucose metabolism led to the contemporary view that impaired pancreatic function determines the development of diabetes. Today, Type 2 diabetes has been classified into over a hundred types and understood as a metabolic disorder characterized by chronically high blood-sugar levels produced by excess caloric intake and lack of physical activity. Type 2 diabetes was formerly known as *adult-onset* diabetes; an earlier iteration was called diabetes mellitus. Similarly, Type 1 diabetes was once referred to as *juvenile* diabetes and earlier, as diabetes insipidus. However, over the last twenty years, changes in diet and lifestyle have had the effect of manifesting adult-onset diabetes in children. Also, better understanding of juvenile-onset diabetes as an autoimmune disease (whereby viral antibodies attack the pancreas) capable of afflicting individuals of any age has resulted in the clinical reclassification of both illnesses as Type 1 and 2 diabetes, respectively. Clinicians I interviewed have diagnosed "adult-onset" (Type 2 diabetes) in three-year-old children and "juvenile-onset" (or Type 1 diabetes) in seventy-year-old adults. These would have been considered medical anomalies fifty years ago. Today they are disconcertingly unremarkable, both in terms of occurrence and comment.

The rising prevalence in Type 2 diabetes in the developing world follows a nearly two-century pattern of urbanization followed by negative nutritional outcomes with obesogenic and diabetogenic consequences.[2] Blood glucose monitoring technology, once confined to the physician's office, today now travels as a portable component of contemporary diabetic life; in the future it may exist in the form of a continuous glucose-monitoring device implanted above the sternum. While the forms these devices take continue to change, their function(ality) remains contested, imperfect, and imprecise. In addition, the interpretation of the numbers they produce in both the professional and lay Type 2 diabetes public continues to drive the redefinition of the illness as well as the patient.

DETECTING SWEETNESS

There are currently three main diabetes diagnostic technologies in clinical use:

1. The hemoglobin (Hb) A1c test reflects serum glucose metabolism over the life of a red blood cell, which is roughly three months. It measures the fraction of metabolized glucose in the hemoglobin. This is known as *glycated* hemoglobin. The normal range for nondiabetics is 4.2–6.0 percent. Diabetes is diagnosed for those above 7.0 percent. *Prediabetes* is reckoned within a liminal diagnostic space of 6.0–7.0 percent.

2. The oral glucose tolerance test (OGTT) measures overnight fasting blood glucose levels and is usually taken in the morning: Diabetes diagnostic benchmark <125 mg/dl.

3. Blood glucose meters (widely known as *glucometers*; commonly referred to as *meters*), used by diabetics to monitor their own blood glucose levels, are also employed in diagnosing diabetes. This deployment is usually reserved for initial assessments in hospital emergency wards, community classes and workshops, and public health screenings. These initial assessments using blood glucometers serve the purpose of detecting individuals with elevated blood glucose levels who can next be referred to the appropriate health care provider. There, she will undergo either the HbA1c test or the OGTT.

The OGTT is considered slightly more reliable than the HbA1c test because, during fasting, glucose in the stored form of glycogen is released from the liver into the blood stream. This is known as the *dawn effect* or *dawn phenomenon*. The dawn effect provides a glucose-rich fasting environment for the OGTT to detect insulin resistance. The OGTT's precise reliability, therefore, is due to its overnight assessment of blood glucose metabolism. But in terms of diagnostic advantage, the HbA1c is considered superior as it measures glucose metabolism over the nearly three-month lifespan of a red blood cell. Further, the OGTT is a clinically based laboratory test, while the HbA1c has the added advantage of being a portable device that can be taken into the field.

In July 2009, the American Diabetes Association's (ADA) Expert Committee issued a position statement concerning the HbA1c and OGTT's comparative accuracy and reliability in diagnosing diabetes. The committee cited the HbA1c test's advantage over the OGTT as

1. providing a better index of overall glycemic exposure and risk for long-term complications,

2. not requiring either fasting or timed samples,
3. having substantially less preanalytic instability,
4. relatively unaffected by acute (e.g., stress- or illness-related) perturbations affecting blood glucose levels, and
5. useful in guiding diabetes management and adjusting therapy.

The expert committee recommended setting the diagnostic threshold for diabetes at 6.5 percent, the level at which elevated blood glucose begins to produce microvascular pathological changes in the retinal structure of the eye.[3] In effect, the sequelae of retinopathy leading to glaucoma constitute one sign of chronically elevated hyperglycemia.

It is unfortunate that T1 and T2 diabetes are both referred to and known as forms of diabetes, given that they have entirely different etiologies and consequences. T1D is the result of an acute viral infection of unknown origin attacking the pancreas and rendering the organ physiologically dysfunctional. Generally speaking, T1 diabetics tend toward low body weight, while obesity figures prominently in both the manifestation and amelioration of Type 2 diabetes. Immediately upon diagnosis, the T1D patient thereafter requires insulin for the rest of their lives. T1D, therefore, is characterized by both its sudden onset and immediate need for insulin. As such, it is also known as insulin-dependent diabetes. What T1D and T2D patients do have in common is the use of blood glucose measurement technologies. However, the T1D patient, who not only requires insulin to live but also tends toward catabolism, or decreasing body weight over time, needs more continuous monitoring. Increasingly, T1 diabetics wear continuous glucose-monitoring devices on waistbands inside their clothes. Some contain insulin pumps that automatically inject insulin into the abdomen of the patient in response to high blood glucose levels at any given time. Others have preset alarms that set off when blood glucose levels either rise or fall beyond acceptable parameters. The use of continuous glucose-monitoring devices and insulin pumps by Type 1 diabetics depends on aesthetics, functional preferences, and affordability. There is a wide price range among this class of blood glucose monitoring devices.

Darlene Pedraza has T1 diabetes. She showed me the continuous glucose monitor taped to her abdomen, equipped with an alarm system that notified her of blood glucose excesses or deficiencies. If in excess, an appropriate dose of insulin is automatically injected into her abdomen; if deficient, she knows to eat a snack with adequate forms of carbohydrate, such as fruit, or better fruit juice, which will be quickly absorbed into the bloodstream. "I wear it 24/7. The thing is, I'm lucky—an insulin pump can cost upwards of nine thousand dollars. If you are on either Medicare or Medi-Cal [Medicaid in California], you can only obtain a pump if you are able to prove that your pancreas is dead." Therefore, in terms of sheer technological and economic disparity, Type 1 diabetics span a much longer continuum of resource inequality than do Type 2 diabetics.

PATHOLOGICAL SWEETNESS

Type 2 diabetics comprise upwards of 95 percent of the entire diabetes population. Type 2 diabetes is amenable to diet and exercise; however, if chronic hyperglycemia is uncontrolled, pharmaceutical interventions along with diet and exercise modifications are attempted. In contrast with T1D, Type 2 diabetes is a slow, progressive illness. Both illnesses can produce multiorgan and systemic pathologies either originating from or exacerbated by chronically elevated blood sugar levels.

While the mechanism by which sweetness becomes pathological remains unclear, in Type 2 diabetes the body still produces insulin, which somehow cannot enter cells and digest glucose. Therefore, Type 2 diabetes is sometimes referred to as *non-insulin-dependent diabetes*. Implicit here is that, unlike Type 1 diabetes, having Type 2 diabetes does not mean that the pancreas is biologically or physiologically "dead." It remains, in most cases, an organ of decreasing regenerative possibility until regeneration becomes no longer possible. At this point, the Type 2 diabetic becomes insulin dependent much like the Type 1 diabetic. Undigested glucose remains in the bloodstream, where it begins adhering to blood vessels, nerve endings, and internal organs. Also, the more body fat accumulated, the more insulin resistant the individual becomes.

Exercise has been demonstrated to draw excess glucose from the blood into the cells, enabling the digestion of glucose (glycolysis) by improving the bioavailability of insulin.[4] If this is truly non-insulin-dependent diabetes, then one would think that increased exercise and improved dietary intake should make both a rational and a practical difference. This chapter examines the historical framing of diabetes

as an illness driven by environmental change, and how that understanding of environmental risk was interpreted subsequently as racial
risk. I offer a narrative history outlining the ways different ethnoracial
groups figured over time into the diabetes research imagination toward exploring the mechanisms driving Type 2 diabetogenesis. In
terms of my wider discussion and broader concern, I show how both
the historical narrative and research imagination have moved inexora-
bly toward African-descent populations.

THE EMERGENCE OF THE THRIFTY GENE

In 1962, James Neel posited that hunter-gatherers possessed a "thrifty
gene" that allowed them to withstand environmental fluctuations and
the vicissitudes of feast and famine in sparse, mostly arid environments. Neel saw "progress" as materially and technologically enabling
a sedentary modern culture living in the midst of caloric abundance.
Populations most recently removed from hunting and gathering, Neel
argued, would be more genetically susceptible to both obesity and diabetes.[5] Neel envisioned diabetes mellitus as an untoward aspect of a
"thriftiness" genotype that is less of an asset today than during the
feast-or-famine days of hunting and gathering cultures. He suggested
the development of specific means to test his hypothesis.[6]

Although he never overtly mentioned race in the article, subsequent
interpretations of Neel's hypothesis racialized his argument, with
southwestern U.S. Native Americans and Latinos with Native American ancestry offered as the model populations of feast-or-famine physiology. So how did Neel's vague hypothesis become a model of racial
specificity, and just when did this interpretive transformation actually
occur?[7] Neel envisioned two future Type 2 diabetes epidemiological
scenarios and the genetic implications of each. Under the unambigu-
ous heading "Some Eugenic Considerations," the first scenario coupled
the globalization of Western diet and cultural practices with advances
in population health. This, Neel argued, would result in an increased
population of individuals with the "thrifty genotype." In the second
scenario, high population pressure resulting in periodic food scarcity
would render the thrifty genotype useful in a similar way that sickle-cell
anemia serves as an evolutionary bioprotective to malaria.[8]

But Neel did not consider whether access to Western medical care
would be available when the rest of world adopted Western patterns

of consumption. Significantly, Neel also did not discuss the value of Western bodies, either to scientific investigation of diabetes risk or the political economy of power that makes for food scarcity and abundance. However, Neel presciently pointed to the potential biovalue of the diabetic genotype by centering on the Other's genetic thriftiness as a desirable biological pool of outstanding genetic material for collection. And, as significant, the research value of the Others' genotype augured potential commercial value for treating Western globalized diabetics.

Neel did not mention the bioethics of collecting this genetic material, or the biopolitics of recruitment, consent, and internal application in diverse, multiethnic societies. Moreover, caloric restriction and increased physical activity also go unremarked in his brief discussion of treatment solutions to the Westernized diabetic body. To his credit, Neel's "Eugenic Considerations" attributed dual bioprotective and biohazardous properties to the thrifty gene based on historical specificities and subsequent environmental adaptations. These historical and environmental "considerations" will figure prominently in later chapters of this book.

While the history of diabetes science often approaches its objects of study from triumphant narrativity and chronological perspectives, I offer an interpretation both against and for Neel's "thrifty-gene" hypothesis: *against,* buttressed by anthropological assertions that race has no biological basis, and *for* in that obesity and Type 2 diabetes represent the contemporary condition of metabolic possibility, or risk, irrespective of "race" or ethnicity—wherever technology and material abundance permit sedentary living in high-caloric environments. In questioning both Neel's original notion of recently sedentized former hunter-gatherers as more susceptible to diabetes and subsequent racial interpretations of diabetic susceptibility, I argue for the universality of the "thrifty gene." In doing so, I seek to make it moot in considering Type 2 diabetic risk. Nevertheless, Neel's hypothesis became part of wider late-twentieth-century conversations about risk and disease, the parameters of prediction and diagnosis, and the ethical politics of research recruitment, with race forming a signal subtext within the scientific narrative. I begin here with a narrative history of diabetic risk and how Neel's racialized risk populations remain indispensable to our discussion of invisible black labor in cardiometabolic research.

FRAMING FRAMINGHAM

Over a decade before Neel's article, the Framingham Study had already begun to examine arteriosclerosis, hypertension, and other risk factors for heart disease among a select group of individuals in Framingham, Massachusetts. While recognizing the desirability of including a more geographically and demographically diverse research population, the study's designers felt that a small town of 25,000–50,000 residents would more than adequately provide the 6,000 adults needed to initiate the research project. In the original article describing the study's rationale, the researchers indicated that they believed a smaller geographic area would make the project more manageable, and the high social capital of the area would make it more efficient in terms of "securing cooperation."[9] They also argued:

> There is, however, reasonable basis for the belief that the distribution of arteriosclerosis and hypertension in the white race in the United States is such that within-community variance is very much greater than between-community variance, and a wide range of type-situations influencing development of these diseases may be found in any community. This hypothesis can only be tested, of course, by similar studies in other communities.[10]

While in principle the Framingham Study researchers valued participatory inclusion, cultural and racial homogeneity were seen as conducive to doing good science. We must remember that in 1951 the civil rights movement had not yet fully taken flight. The politics of inclusion were still more than a decade away, while the bioethics of inclusion remained a longer-term project, as Tuskegee and other experiments continued and as Henrietta Lacks's cervical cancer cells were about to create medical history.[11]

Yet in their statement, the Framingham scientists hint at three important points. First, the argument that greater diversity exists within groups than between groups was, in 1951, conceptually ahead of anthropological notions of difference at the time; that realization would have to wait for Edmund Leach's groundbreaking work in far-away Burma.[12] Second, in arguing for greater in-group diversity, the researchers presaged the metabolic contingency Neel would later pose in this thrifty-gene hypothesis, which, as I read it, asserted a physiological metabolic contingency, not a racial metabolic contingency, an argument that diaspora alone, for example, cannot account for. I make this interpretation of Neel despite his possible intention in formulating his hypothesis, which in short, neither presumed correlations between race and risk, nor, by implication, between race and biology. That said, both the Framingham researchers and Neel were careful not to reify race in formulating and articulating an explanatory language of obesity, Type 2 diabetes, and cardiometabolic risk. Both imagined populations of environmental, not racial, difference. So how, in the case of Type 2 diabetes, did the African American, Latino, Native American, and Jewish body become the wrong body of risk to inherit, but the right body for clinical research, diabetes education, and public health stakeholders?

DO THE (LATINO) EYES HAVE IT?

While undergoing a routine eye examination at the University of California, Berkeley, School of Optometry, I was asked by the chief ophthalmologist about my research. Having just returned from New York after fieldwork in the summer and fall of 2009, I desperately needed a fresh set of lenses through which to see the next phase of my project. When I responded that I was interested in the interplay between Type 2 diabetic risk and technology, he asked if I had heard of the Los Angeles Latino Eye Study. When I said no, he confided in me that eye examinations there at the optometry school had also been uncovering a surprising number of cases of prediabetic retinopathy among Latino students, staff, and faculty associated with the university.

The Los Angeles Latino Eye Study (LALES) was based on a cohort of 6,357 individuals recruited from six areas of Los Angeles. The study's objective aimed at developing "a population-based assessment of the prevalence of visual impairment, ocular disease, and visual functioning in Latinos."[13] In contrast with the ADA's Expert Committee recommendation of a 6.5 percent diabetic diagnostic threshold, the LA Latino Eye Study noted initial retinal pathology occurring in individuals with hemoglobin A1c readings of 6.0 percent. Although intense debate remains in clinical circles as to what the diagnostic threshold should be, confusion also remains as to what HbA1c level constitutes successful therapeutic blood glucose control in existing diabetics. Many clinicians and diabetes educators see an HbA1c reading of <7.0 percent as a successful blood glucose control target. However, both the ADA's Expert Committee's 6.5 percent recommended diagnostic threshold and the new retinoscopic technologies detecting prediabetic retinopathy in individuals with HbA1c readings as low as 6.0 percent highlight the interplay between technology and interpretation, as it was found that intensive pharmaceutical treatment of those between 6.0 and 7.0 percent resulted in increased risk of mortality.[14]

The study's authors cautioned against "automatically applying" the research's conclusions to other Latino groups. Despite this caveat, it urged replicative studies among other Latino groups based on the assumption that "Additional data on these Latino subgroups will help provide insight into the similarity of the prevalence of eye disease in these populations."[15] Interestingly, the statement infers an ethnoracial category generative of objective truth about that group, however admittedly diverse that subpopulation's members, inviting sweeping generalizations that call into question racial categorization as a reliable biological descriptor and index of risk.

This was reflected in the Latino Eye Study final report. The term "Latino" was used in making claims about "Latino" rates of diabetic retinopathy, despite the fact that all the Latinos in the study were "mainly of Mexican descent" living in La Puente, California.[16] The report repeatedly posed Latino risk numbers in comparison with white risk numbers, reinscribing race and risk through the discursive and scientific use of poorly defined, almost arbitrarily viewed, ethnoracial categories. While tangentially instructive, I suggest that the LA Latino Eye Study's primary value resides in understanding and addressing the needs of the community in La Puente as well as wider Mexican/American/Chicano diasporic and transnational communities. Such research will expose more socioeconomic, psychological, and other environmental factors at play than any inherently biological fault lines in the seismic study of diabetes.

THE EMERGENCE OF THE AT-RISK NATIVE AMERICAN DIABETIC

A series of post–World War II films produced by the U.S. Indian Bureau (later the Bureau of Indian Affairs) depicted two groups of Native Americans, the Pima and Havasupai.[17] Both films portrayed vibrant, healthy, and active communities. The 1946 film about the Havasupai offered bucolic scenes displaying the traditional forms of farming, food preservation, and material culture of a seemingly autonomous group living in relative isolation at the bottom of the Grand Canyon. The 1948 Pima film, directed and filmed by F. C. Clark Jr., is a "story based on a report by Irrigation Engineer C. H. Southworth."[18] It fails to mention that the tribe's water sources had been diverted, not for the benefit of the Pima but for white farmers who had colonized the area over the previous three quarters of a century.

Behind the orchestrated appearances lay a metabolic time bomb that was gradually eroding the health of both tribes. The Potemkin-esque representations of Pima and Havasupai self-sufficiency obfuscated processes of resource dispossession occurring in their midst, processes by which they were becoming dependent upon external sources for foods such as white flour, sugar, lard, canned foods, and coffee. Both films romanticized the struggle of survival narratively within the circumscribed and easily policed perimeters of tradition and culture, a struggle amenable to victory through Western technological advancement and rational political organization.

The geographic isolation of the Pima and Havasupai, combined with subsequently increasing rates of obesity and Type 2 diabetes, and perhaps most importantly, their relative genetic homogeneity, made each group successive targets of the diabetes research gaze. While the Pima have the highest rate of Type 2 diabetes in the world, they are among the most studied.[19] The Havasupai on the other hand, live in a more geographically secluded area than the Pima, and have, relatively, only more recently come under research scrutiny.[20] What new understandings could William Blake's "America" offer the body of "Europe," and by moral extension of the Enlightenment's promise, "the World?"

From 1990 to 1994, researchers from Arizona State University collected blood samples from members of the Havasupai to study diabetes and other cardiometabolic disorders within the group. Later, it was found that Havasupai genetic material was not used for the research purposes intended and agreed to previously with the Human Subjects/Internal Review Board at Arizona State University.[21] The Havasupai filed suit, seeking US$75 million in damages. In the 2010 case *Arizona State Board of Regents v. Havasupai Tribe*, it was revealed that some of the collected blood samples were used for research into schizophrenia and the effects of inbreeding on the tribe. PhD dissertations were written by and degrees awarded to individuals who based their work on the misappropriated genetic material; the material was even used by senior researchers as well.[22]

In the end, the tribe settled for $700,000, citing satisfaction with having secured a moral victory.[23] Yet while the Havasupai could claim a moral victory, it remains uncertain as to whether any prescriptive ethical framework for future research recruitment emerged from the case. Institutionally, no dissertations were voided, PhD degrees revoked, or senior researchers adversely affected professionally as an outcome of the court's decision. The relative genetic and geographic isolation of a diabetes-ravaged population proved as enticing a research body of contrapuntal difference as the genetic diversity of sub-Saharan populations would in the future, albeit to an inverse degree.

The specificities of biological change resulting from shifting historical and cultural practices have added new variables that challenge notions of comparable racial categories. Representations of historically shaped black bodies, coded as "property," occupy a socioeconomic position subordinated to historically shaped white bodies, coded as "owners."[24] Furthermore, the legacy experience of African Americans as commoditized and insured individual units of monetized property backed by legal sanction differs in significant ways from the idea of "possession" when referring to Indigeneity. *Terra nullius*, or "empty land," placed value on and rationalized the appropriation of Native American lands and resources, but not their labor.[25] Nevertheless, the idea of race as a relevant category of differentiated biological value continues in genomic and postgenomic research, posing new questions about the permeability of the nature/culture divide in articulating accurate estimations of biological difference and risk.[26]

The case of the Havasupai reflected the ongoing historical project represented by Blake's "America" in bonded service to the care of "Europe" as life itself. Yet over the course of the second-half of the twentieth century, "Africa" would become the next imagined body of Type 2 biosecrets.

THE EMERGENCE OF THE AFRICAN AMERICAN DIABETIC

As Arlene Tuchman has noted, one hundred years ago conventional medical wisdom viewed diabetes as a mainly "Jewish" disease. At that time, blacks were seen as a low-risk diabetes population, with Jews framed problematically as a high-risk "racial" group.[27] Tuchman argues that diabetes risk among Jews had less to do with racial biology than an increasingly sedentized and affluent U.S. urban lifestyle among an immigrant population with largely impoverished Eastern European origins—hardly Neel's new conscripts to modernity recently removed from hunting and gathering. Today, neither public health nor clinical science has taken lessons from, or much less remembers, their respective historical attempts at linking Jewish ancestry with Type 2 diabetes susceptibility. In the absence of this historical reflexivity concerning contemporary methodological approaches equating race and biology, African Americans and other minority groups currently garner global research recruitment attention as featured high-risk diabetes populations.[28]

Around the turn of the twentieth century, colonial physicians in West Africa remarked on the rarity of diabetes among native Africans, attributing this to their high-fiber, low-animal-protein diet, replete with a diverse intake of fruit and vegetables.[29] Similarly, it was said that although "Negroes" in the West Indies lived closer to fresh produce and nature's bounty, the benefits disappeared upon immigrating to New York City, manifesting subsequently with a 98 percent prevalence of rickets in that population. The change to a more devitalized diet, along with a marked decrease in sun exposure, contributed to the development both of vitamin D deficiency and the increased risk of Type 2 diabetes.[30]

At the end of World War I, Army physicians reported the near absence of diabetes among African American soldiers, in stark contrast with white soldiers. In a cowritten report by the U.S. Marine Corps and the U.S. Sanitary Corps using data collected for the Report of the Surgeon General of the U.S. Army in 1918, the authors concluded that although African American soldiers suffered more than white soldiers from respiratory and venereal diseases, as well as from both smallpox and chicken pox, they contracted diabetes at half the rate. They summarized:

> The colored troops are relatively less resistant to diseases of
> the lungs and pleura as well as to certain general diseases, like
> tuberculosis and smallpox; they are also much more frequently
> infected with venereal diseases and suffer widespread complica-
> tions of these diseases. But the uninfected negro is highly resistant

to diseases of the skin, mouth and throat. He seems to have
more stable nerves, has better eyes and metabolizes better. Thus,
in many respects the uninfected colored troops show themselves
to be constitutionally better physiological machines than the
white men.[31]

While the authors concluded that "uninfected" African American soldiers were "better physiological machines than the white men," full
inclusion in the U.S. armed services would take another World War
to bring about. This subpopulation was not then seen as metabolically
compromised, as often assumed today, but quite the opposite, if only
to scientifically validate the biopolitical utility of African Americans
for military service. As for the "infected," what went unremarked in
the report was the unequal to nonexistent medical care in these soldiers' communities of origin and civilian residence.[32] History would
later show "the infected" proving more valuable as research subjects
than as citizens deserving of timely and appropriate treatment. This
future bioethical breach would have far-reaching implications for the
future recruitment of African Americans in bioscientific research trials
and overall sense of trust in the medical system. Although the category
African American was not socially or politically embraced until the
early to mid-1980s, the increased media spotlight over roughly the last
four decades demonstrates the heightened visibility and centrality of
African Americans in both the popular media and scientific research
gazes. The category "black" continues to have definitional traction, as
the terms *African American, African immigrant, Afro-Caribbean,* and so
on continue to arouse contested debates surrounding identity, culture,
and difference within and without diasporic and transnational actors,
groups, and networks.[33]

Framingham researchers identified the white, middle-class citizen
as the universal research subject most amenable to universal scientific
rationality. What went unmarked was the categorical construction of
"white" in the research imagination and the conceptual and methodological implications such crude categorical efforts would have on the
organization of other "races" within the inclusive research future the
authors urged. While aware of the flaws and limitations of this categorical approach, they nevertheless encouraged future research among diverse populations. Yet, implicit in the selection of the Framingham
Study site and participants remained the unanswered question of en-

vironment as a desirable and important research variable in examining culturally unknown populations, those "alien but not exotic fellow citizens" stratified by education, class, and geography, and crosscut by socialized gender and racial constructs. The intersectionality of these different elemental social constructs has gained research and, as this book will explore in later chapters, market valence since 1951.[34]

REFRAMING FRAMINGHAM

I present the Framingham Study in this book for two important reasons. First, it marked the initial research-recruitment foray into the science of establishing measurable biomarkers for predicting risk occurrence in arteriosclerosis, heart disease, and hypertension, illnesses comprising what later became part of what is now called the cardiometabolic syndrome (MetS).[35] This syndrome encompasses a constellation of conditions, including obesity, hyperlipidemia, hypertension, hyperglycemia, renal disease, eye-disease retinopathy, and nerve-damaging neuropathy. More recently, Alzheimer's disease has been included as part of the syndrome. The combination of these conditions has a negative effect on cardiovascular health, hence the term *cardiometabolic syndrome*. Second, as Type 2 diabetes is now a recognized component of the cardiometabolic illness constellation, Framingham serves as the conceptual and methodological antecedent that further contextualizes Neel's later argument: Type 2 diabetics are prone to developing heart disease and kidney disease, arteriosclerosis, and hypertension, and inversely, people with cardiometabolic disorders have higher chances of developing Type 2 diabetes.

Both Framingham and Neel have since been read through racial and other lenses, in concert with Du Bois's observation nearly a century ago that explanatory claims about the inherent biology of certain racial and ethnic groups shift based on the theoretical and scientific notions of the day.[36] Mid-twentieth-century science misappropriated the thrifty-gene hypothesis to incorrectly explain obesity in various Native American and Latino groups.[37] Since Framingham and Neel, these, along with the case of the Havasupai and Pima in Arizona, raise questions about the morality and ethics of racial and ethnic correlations and associations about Type 2 diabetes causation and prevalence.

In addition, tellingly, and most instructive moving forward in this book, the Framingham researchers in 1951 presciently defined and included cardiometabolic illnesses as *epidemic,* an ascription that today has been extended to obesity and Type 2 diabetes.[38] Such an ascription implies no racial causation, correlation, or selective risk. *Epidemics* (*over* the *demos,* or people) are characterized by an illness or disease occurrence that moves impartially across geographic space through various demographic groups. *Endemic* (*within* the *demos*) is defined as an illness or disease originating and occurring within a specific place or group, sui generis—a reproducible pathological manifestation in either geographic or phenotypic isolation. *Pandemic* (*across* the *demos*) is defined as an illness or disease originating and occurring within multiple locales simultaneously. Therefore, in delinking race from risk, I argue that obesity, Type 2 diabetes, and other cardiometabolic disorders are epidemic, endemic, and pandemic today.[39]

Although racial and ethnic recruitment did not figure prominently in early diabetes biomedical and biotechnological science, larger cardiometabolic research foci based on race have increased in research valence over the last fifty years since Neel's oeuvre. I take none of these categories (race, diabetes, and risk) for granted in recounting how researchers, medical providers, public health professionals, and community groups have circulated them discursively. These three categories—race, diabetes, and risk—generate a coproductive instability rather than the assumption of any steady classificatory state. Indeed, it was the productive ambiguity of the contested prediabetes classification that enabled the pharmaceutical turn and heightened the desire for African-descent participation in Type 2 diabetes biotechnological research.

FRAMING AMBIGUITY: PREDIABETES PREDICTION AND THE PHARMACEUTICAL TURN

Prediabetes is a technologically ascertainable, yet subjectively asymptomatic index of Type 2 diabetic risk. According to the Centers for Disease Control (CDC), as of 2014, approximately eighty-six million prediabetics existed in the United States. Inclusive of diagnosed diabetics, over 40 percent of these individuals remained undiagnosed.[40] Although technological advances have allowed a certain imprecise accuracy in measuring blood glucose levels, the matter of interpretation remains central to this discussion.

Prediabetes is based on "arbitrary" diagnostic values due to its ambiguous intermediacy.[41] Since the turn of the century, doctors have increasingly recommended early and aggressive pharmaceutical intervention in the treatment of prediabetes.[42] Further, the classificatory boundaries of Type 2 diabetes have expanded through both pharmaceutical market logics and diagnostic technological advances.[43] The clinical gaze aligned with pharmaceutical company visions, and how both (re)informed changing classificatory categories of diabetes deserves particular attention. But first, I want to contextualize this discussion within a larger medical history concerning Type 2 diabetes predictive risk, prediabetes, and the technologies that enable their measurement.

In the 1970s, a handful of medical studies linked obesity, glucose tolerance, and insulin response under the clinical term *protodiabetes*. The *protodiabetic* was seen as an individual, usually obese, demonstrating impaired fasting-glucose levels and reduced insulin response in the absence of diabetes.[44] The *prediabetic* on the other hand, was also defined as someone having impaired fasting-glucose levels and reduced insulin response, in addition to impaired pancreatic beta-cell and liver functioning.[45] As early as 1974, research began to show a strong correlation between weight loss and improved insulin response in the protodiabetic.[46] Although the term *prediabetes* had been used since the 1960s, the term was seen as crude and inexact: *potential, latent,* and *early* diabetics were seen as better descriptors of what were then considered complex physiological processes.[47]

Recent genetic ascriptions of chronic disease causality have found fertile ground for research in the Caribbean.[48] The thrifty-gene hypothesis, along with other racialized genetic tropes, is being proffered as the basis for understanding the high prevalence of diabetes, hypertension, and obesity in the region.[49] However, little ethnographic attention has been made between state, corporate, and citizen social actors in the Caribbean concerning pharmaceutical interventions for these chronic illnesses.

Given these lacunae in the literature, Ian Whitmarsh extended Michel Laguerre's notion of "rejected knowledge" (in situating Caribbean local medical epistemologies within the context of colonial medical and evaluative social structures and praxes) to include local forms of biomedical praxis and national biopolitical objectives that contest the biomarket grammar and hype of international pharmaceutical regimes.[50] Whitmarsh's article "Biomedical Ambivalence: Asthma Diagnosis, the

Pharmaceutical, and other Contradictions in Barbados" focuses ethnographic attention as to how "rejected biomedical knowledge" is embedded within local forms of biopolitical control as well as postcolonial diagnostic mimesis of the medical/pharmaceutical metropole. Whitmarsh's subsequent book-length ethnographic examination of asthma diagnosis in Barbados questions ascribed racial categories from the United States and their epistemic slippages between biological and social notions of race.[51] NIH and FDA racial categories travel and in turn inform racial identity on this slippery biological and social terrain. Whitmarsh gives attention to how North Atlantic research epistemologies, methodologies, and praxes sought to accommodate themselves in Barbados, and the liminal spaces they created. I borrow here Sarah Franklin's use of the "liminal" space to trace how "life" is redefined and reinterpreted.[52] More precisely, how do the creation of biological properties "reveal specific national and economic priorities, moral and civic values, and technoscientific institutional cultures?"[53] Stakeholders reify these medical categories: physicians, families, and the state are all imbricated in these truth claims around disease and national medical sovereignty in ways that simultaneously aspire to and reject North Atlantic putative norms and labels.

I find Franklin useful in reading Whitmarsh's ethnographic examination of how Creole science and medicine is constructed.[54] In this case, the marketed cultivation of new medical and social epistemes, ontologies, and praxes crystallizes around an ambiguous and contested entity (i.e., *the symptom, race, the science, biostatistics, the diagnosis,* etc.) within a powerful imagined (cultural, national, or therapeutic) future. It evokes Lucy Suchman's concern about how the "relentless normativity" of technoscientific engagement flattens social topography by the virtue of its claimed objective/impartial rationality.[55]

For our purposes moving forward, Whitmarsh provokes several important questions:

> How are local bodies rendered amenable to biopharmaceutical recruitment, research and treatment, and do both local physicians and national institutions of health serve as interlocutors for this biopolitical/capital process? How is "inclusion" desired, constructed, contested, or perhaps even unavoidable?[56] How is expertise assessed and what are its methods of interpretation?

Can expertise be located within the local, or is it an accretive, international practice? Are the local and the national even relevant socio-spatial categories, or do they refract intra- and extra- institutional relationships to power, knowledge, and capital? And inversely, how are these technologically mediated forms of categorical ascription and analysis networked and con-structed in the medical/scientific metropole itself?[57]

While Whitmarsh's article's title accurately points toward ambiva-lence, he creates valuable theoretical tension by counterpositioning ambivalence with ambiguity. It should be noted that his article is en-titled "Biomedical Ambivalence" but his book is entitled "Biomedical Ambiguity." However, he never truly differentiates between the two. This poses important methodological, analytical, and even ethical questions in terms of how the ethnographer attempts to "translate" contradiction, incommensurability, emergent biopolitical and bio-capital assemblages of technological surveillance, and new regimes of citizen/consumer/patient-hood. Ambiguity and ambivalence are neither synonymous nor metonymous; they each occupy different moral and epistemological terrains reflecting differing forms of intent and deployment on the ground. Whitmarsh grapples with the metho-dological problematic of translation, yet given the stakes involved (particularly as posed later in this book), I am left wondering whether either ambivalence or ambiguity productively push the interrogation far enough. Framing ambiguity, even productive and profitable ambi-guity such as in the cases of prediabetes and racial classification, pre-sents a difficult exercise in locating and situating their parametric risk boundaries due to their definitional instability.

DIAGNOSING PREDIABETIC AMBIGUITY

To this point, in the second decade of the twenty-first century, de-termining a firm Type 2 diabetes diagnostic threshold continues to arouse debate in both clinical and public health circles. Technological advances in recent years have complicated efforts to understand its precursor, prediabetes, in terms of actionable risk or treatable illness. In 2001, the Biomarkers Working Group at the NIH defined a *bio-marker* as "a biological molecule found in blood, other bodily fluids, or tissue which represents a sign of a normal or abnormal process or of a condition or disease. A biomarker may be used to see how well the body responds to a treatment for a disease or condition."[58]

However, in a 2010 position paper, the ADA shied away from the term *prediabetes* and its implications that biomarkers of a presymptomatic stage of diabetes had been found. In their view, intermediate diagnostic values represent a high risk for the future development of Type 2 diabetes, signaling heightened susceptibility to developing a range of cardiometabolic illnesses such as hypertension and heart disease. Despite this rhetorical shift to "intermediate diagnostic values," what the authors termed "categories of increased risk" were seen as warranting biomedical intervention just as much as the term *prediabetes.*[59] Early research demonstrated the malleability of protodiabetes as both an illness category and physiological contingency in the face of improved dietary and lifestyle changes, and resultant weight loss. Today, *prediabetes* has been classified according to what was formerly termed *protodiabetes.* In effect, the time of progression to the condition and imagined pathways forward has shifted from prevention to treatment.

In the field, I heard different views concerning these new interpretations of prediabetes and the new treatment protocols they attempt to rationalize. At a diabetes-education class in the Livermore Valley, a prediabetic individual asked Darlene Pedraza, "When should I know to begin 'pampering' my liver with Metformin?" Metformin, the most prescribed drug in newly diagnosed cases of Type 2 diabetes, was now being prescribed to prediabetics. Surprisingly, Darlene Pedraza responded by calling the notion of prediabetes as pathology a "theory." Her recommendation: "Evaluate your own personal and familial risk for diabetes, then go talk to your doctor about whether your condition necessitates pharmaceutical therapy. You never know, you might just end up bringing them new information."

As a practical matter, the notion of prediabetes as a theory on the one hand and as a contingent fact on the other both ring true in the case of Type 2 diabetes risk. In contrast with Darlene's statement just mentioned, a public health official I interviewed viewed the situation differently. We had been discussing the rationale behind the pharmaceuticalization of prediabetes. Although diet and lifestyle alone have been shown to prevent prediabetic progression to Type 2 diabetes, Darren cited the inability of large numbers of patients to manifest the necessary behavioral shifts required in making diet and lifestyle changes therapeutically effective. Also, in his view, contemporary obesity complicates the issue entirely. In the case of both diagnosed prediabetes and predicted Type 2 diabetes risk, "We must," in his words, "treat patients within the context of their lives."

TESTING CONTEXTS: DIET, LIFESTYLE, AND METFORMIN

From 1996 to 1999, the Diabetes Prevention Program (DPP), the most ambitious diabetes research project to date, recruited over three thousand volunteers with impaired glucose tolerance (IGT). In terms of aim, size, scope, and longitudinal continuity, the DPP is the diabetes research equivalent of the Framingham Study's cardiometabolic focus. The research volunteers, technically prediabetic, were evaluated and selected primarily by the fasting oral glucose tolerance test. Involving over twenty medical centers and research teams, the project's four control groups—Metformin, Intensive Lifestyle Modification, Placebo, and Troglitazone—were examined to measure the onset of Type 2 diabetes in these four groups of individuals with IGT.[60] Essentially an efficacy trial, the DPP was envisioned as providing a basis for more informed prevention and treatment strategies.[61]

The results of the DPP clearly demonstrated the superiority of intensive lifestyle modification (diet, exercise, stress reduction) in preventing the onset of Type 2 diabetes over a longer ten-year period than either the Metformin or Placebo groups. More important to our later discussion, over the shorter term of less than five years, lifestyle change and Metformin were equally effective in preventing T2D onset.[62] Both Darlene and Darren understand the contexts in people's lives that prevent quick adoption of diet and lifestyle modifications in the face of a Type 2 diagnosis, much less prediabetes. Herself a Type 1 diabetic, Darlene adheres to an active fitness program and vegetarian diet. But, as she explained,

> Some physicians and clinicians don't understand why diabetics, and especially prediabetic patients, don't make lifestyle changes faster, in light of the evidence that these changes can make a big difference. They almost see it as a simple self-discipline and self-control issue. A lot of these folks [physicians and clinicians], and I've seen it, are highly disciplined people who developed or

already had these habits during their professional education. They can't understand why everybody can't get up at 4:30 every morning and exercise before working a twelve-hour day like they do. But these are proactive Type As who have been successful with most things they've tried. And most of them don't have diabetes.

While Darlene recognizes the importance of diet and lifestyle, personally and professionally, she was careful in tailoring her diabetes message to her audience. Her comment implied that some physicians and clinicians make a moral connection between behavior and success. Self-control as a means of successfully determining desired outcomes comes easier to some than to others, and often carries with it moral connotations, something the successful need remember in counseling those they see as lacking in self-discipline and willpower. Yet Darlene's comment further suggests the unique challenges that diabetics face, challenges much different and ultimately more consuming than the life hurdles routinely cleared by diabetes experts and clinicians without diabetes.

Currently, there are three treatment options for reducing obesity and improving glucose metabolism: diet, exercise, and lifestyle change; pharmaceutical regimens; and, bariatric, or gastric bypass surgery. Children tend to respond better to diet, exercise, and lifestyle change, and adults to drug therapy. Bariatric surgery produces the fastest weight loss; however, permanent results vary, and further, many of these individuals disperse into the general population leaving no data trail to evaluate.[63] A recent ADA Position Paper on Nutrition found exercise to contribute only modestly to weight loss, while improving insulin sensitivity and long-term health maintenance. Exercise proved most successful when combined with behavioral-modification therapy. The authors could find no consistent nutritional guidelines for healthy weight loss, and macronutrient requirements have not yet been developed. Interestingly, the authors claim greater success with antiobesity medication than either diet or exercise in those with body mass indexes (BMI) >27.0. They argued that dietary regimens consistently fell prey to weight regain, although exercise was seen as a useful long-term strategy, but too slow to make an effective therapeutic intervention in the obese patient either at high risk for or with Type 2 diabetes.[64] It appears that within the contexts of peoples' lives, obese adults respond better to pharmacotherapy than lifestyle interventions.

But with pharmaceutical intervention, where does prevention end and treatment begin? And when—in the liminal prediabetic or diagnosed diabetic condition?

I use the word *intervention* here due to clinical uncertainty as to whether introduced pharmaceutical regimens should be considered *treatment* of prediabetes, as *therapy,* or *prevention* of diabetes, as *prophylaxis.* Various meta-analyses have been conducted to determine the efficacy of introduced pharmaceutical interventions in addressing prediabetes. The rationale undergirding these interventions aims at preventing the onset of full-blown Type 2 diabetes. However, three arguments have already been proven: First, a 2004 study established the effectiveness of dietary and lifestyle change over pharmaceutical intervention in delaying Type 2 diabetes onset within a three-year period.[65] Second, it is already known that 80 percent of prediabetics can normalize their blood sugar levels through diet and lifestyle interventions alone.[66] Third, Type 2 diabetes patients who meet the American Heart Association's (AHA) weekly aerobic exercise targets and dietary recommendations can sharply reduce, if not eliminate, their dependence on medication.[67] More boldly, the Physicians Committee for Responsible Medicine (PCRM) argues that following a high-fiber, complex-carbohydrate-based, vegan diet can reduce if not eliminate pharmaceutical interventions for Type 2 diabetes.[68]

Even with uncertainty as to whether pharmaceutical interventions control blood glucose levels or impede the (inevitable) Type 2 diabetes process, pharmaceutical approaches are being promoted over diet and lifestyle change in the prediabetic individual. *Pharmaceutical approaches* or *pharmaceutical interventions* perhaps best describe these new prediabetes drug protocols, as the indeterminacy of the illness category raises the question as to whether this constitutes prevention or treatment.[69] Moreover, these marketed pharmaceutical regimes reveal intricate ties both to the technologies that produce them as well as to those clinical technologies that rationalize their prescription.

Risk prediction and diagnostic technologies occupy the "middle rung" of biotechnology market profitability, between "low-ticket" medical commodities with relatively low development cost and profit margins, such as surgical procedures and associated technologies, and "high-ticket" pharmaceutical drug development and sales.[70] Bariatric surgery results in drastic weight loss and often in a reversal of Type 2 diabetes and the consequent elimination of the need for medication.[71]

Even though bariatric surgery costs more than pharmaceutical therapy and diet/lifestyle interventions, patients were more successful in
keeping weight off than with the two former approaches, and experienced more quality-of-life years as well.[72] In short, bariatric patients
received more bang for their diabetic buck.

Such is the case with prediabetes. As one public health official related to me in 2009, "For all intents and purposes, prediabetes is now a
separate disease category requiring aggressive intervention. Advances
in diagnostic technology have made this determination possible."

THE POLITICS OF PRECISION

Clinical research has shown that pharmaceutical attempts at lowering
HbA1c to the "prediabetic" control threshold of <7.0 percent carries
its own risks. The purpose of these research efforts was to examine
whether pharmaceutically induced intensive blood glucose control
had a positive effect on reducing cardiovascular complications and
outcomes. The results were less than impressive.

Because of ongoing uncertainty regarding whether intensive glycemic control can reduce the increased risk of cardiovascular disease
(CVD) in people with Type 2 diabetes, several large long-term trials
were launched in the past decade. These trials compare the effects of intensive and standard glycemic control on CVD outcomes in relatively
high-risk participants with established Type 2 diabetes. In 2008, two of
these trials, Action in Diabetes and Vascular Disease—Preterax and
Diamicron Modified Release Controlled Evaluation (ADVANCE)
and the Veterans Affairs Diabetes Trial (VADT), were completed and
showed no significant reduction in cardiovascular outcomes with intensive glycemic control.[73]

However, previous research showed a positive correlation between
intensive glycemic control and adverse cardiovascular outcomes. In
1961, the University Group Diabetes Program (UGDP) sought to test
the efficacy of tolbutamide, a sulfonyurea drug, in the treatment of
Type 2 diabetes. The UGDP, a research collaborative founded by Max
Miller of Case Western University and Harvey Knowles of the University of Cincinnati, completed its recruitment of volunteers in 1966,
and continued until 1975. Throughout, the UGDP encountered criticism from two opposing factions: diabetes clinicians and the pharmaceutical industry. Clinical diabetes communities initially doubted the

suitability of the drug, while the Upjohn Company paid academics, researchers, and biostatisticians to attack the UGDP program in defense of tolbutamide, which it produced under the brand name Orinase.[74]

Another trial, the 2008 Action to Control Cardiovascular Risk in Diabetes (ACCORD) was discontinued after the discovery that the project's aggressive pharmaceutical strategy of reducing HbA1c levels to <6.0 percent resulted in increased mortality among research participants.[75] To put this into perspective, the LA Latino Eye Study found microvascular pathologies occurring in individuals with an HbA1c level of <6.0 percent, well within the normally accepted range of successful blood glucose control of <7.0 percent, but below the ADA diabetes diagnostic threshold of 6.5 percent. These three studies raised questions as to both the role of intensive pharmaceutical blood glucose control as well as the prospects for reducing cardiovascular complications without iatrogenically producing (or drug inducing) negative cardiovascular outcomes. Ethnicity, HbA1c diagnostic thresholds, and treatment now intersected, nuancing notions of universal diagnostic standardization and treatment indications.

As a result of these ambiguous trial findings, in 2009, three organizations that have historically been less than collaborative—the ADA, the American College of Cardiology (ACC), and the AHA—decided to reevaluate the clinical recommendations for targeted blood glucose levels for diabetics.[76] Realizing that aggressive pharmaceutical blood-glucose-lowering strategies increased cardiovascular mortality, the three major organizations jointly recommended a comprehensive treatment approach to the entire cardiometabolic constellation of illnesses. They did not advise attempting to lower HbA1c levels below 7.0 percent but recommended diet, lifestyle, aspirin use, and so on as important synergistic elements of a total treatment program.[77]

However, by 2018, the HbA1c controversy resurfaced. This time, the American College of Physicians (ACP) and the American Association of Clinical Endocrinologists/American College of Endocrinology (AACE/ACE) offered their own but dissimilar target HbA1c guidelines. The ACP argued for a target range of 7.0–8.0 percent, while the AACE/ACE suggested HbA1c targets of ≤6.5 percent.[78] The ADA continued its recommendation of an effective control target of <7.0 percent.[79]

The earlier DPP, ADVANCE, VADT, and ACCORD trials found that intensive blood glucose control worked best with those who were both younger and had had diabetes for a relatively short time.[80] Given the curve between when aggressive pharmaceutical intervention proves harmful or beneficial, and the emphasized importance of a comprehensive cardiovascular approach, one begins to see the constraining limits of drug therapy and the sustainable potential of diet and lifestyle changes. The safest way to lower one's blood glucose level is through exercise and diet; the majority of the cardiovascular mortalities in the ACCORD study were due to drug-induced (iatrogenic) hypoglycemia. As a further point of emphasis, it should be noted here that all three studies (ADVANCE, VADT, ACCORD) were drug studies; none had an independent diet and/or lifestyle component included in its blood glucose control research protocol.

OF CONTEXTS AND CONTROVERSY

The 2018 controversy reignited debate over the benefits of intensive blood glucose control and the risk of increased cardiovascular mortality from such an approach. It settled neither, while highlighting the ACP's more relaxed guidelines as its recognition of the real life struggles that people with the illness must cope with daily. As we near the end of the second decade of the century, both the early and late stages of Type 2 diabetes onset continue to respond better to cardiovascular-friendly activities, foods, and molecules (such as aspirin) than through a tunnel-vision pharmaceutical approach that sees "successful" blood glucose control as the Holy Grail of diabetes therapy and management. Darlene Pedraza's ambiguity over the science of prediabetes is based on the knowledge that diet and lifestyle changes remain the best long-term, sustainable, and healthy way of living with the ambiguous uncertainties of Type 2 diabetes and its debilitating and often-fatal cardiometabolic consequences. The "contexts of people's lives" alluded to earlier make therapeutic room for those who need that five-year progress-to-illness window established by the Diabetes Prevention Program to make necessary life changes before associated cardiometabolic pathologies begin to alter living contexts for the worse. As an efficacy trial, the DPP sought to apply the basic science of molecular chemistry and physiological systematics solely within a clinical research setting. However, in terms of real-world *effectiveness*, the DPP fell short in terms of enunciating improved therapeutic *effi-*

cacy by making available and circulating new knowledge about both Type 2 diabetes and its treatment.

"Contexts," like "diasporas," vary in terms of disparities in access, cultural competence, technological forms of socialized inertia, environmental health and social justice, and medical literacy, among other factors. The results of the UGDP, DPP, ACCORD, ADVANCE, and VADT trials brought to light competing and collaborative professional and economic rationales shaping both Type 2 diabetes public-health outreach and research recruitment. The arguably belated collaboration between the ADA, ACC, and the AHA, and later disagreements between the ACP, AACE/ACE, the ADA and others, exposed similar professional and economic fault lines: the ongoing professional politics of clinical standardization of HbA1c levels represent, pragmatically, millions if not billions of dollars in pharmaceutical company profits or losses for every percentage of recommended target goals.[81]

However, ambiguity—whether concerning diabetes classification, the role of lifestyle and pharmaceutical interventions, or diagnostic imprecision—intersects constructions of race and risk, and runs rife through this chapter and into the next. The history of prediabetes and diabetes, originally not premised upon racial or ethnic notions of or correlations with Type 2 diabetes risk or prevalence, has increasingly focused on racial theories of risk over the course of the twentieth century and into the twenty-first.[82] The five- and ten-year window to diabetes onset established by the DPP provided clinical and market space to predict diabetes risk, while relying on older ethnoracial constructs in developing ostensibly neutral algorithms of risk. The next chapter takes up the case of one biotechnology company's efforts at racial recruitment to argue that race does not perform reliably as biology, by illustrating how such an approach failed recruitment, clinical, and consequential market challenges.

3

Algorithms of Risk and Race

RECRUITING BLACK RISK AND
MARKETING BLACK BODIES

Be able to tell your patients they are at risk for diabetes
before their bodies do.

—Tethys BioSciences Advertisement

In June 2009 at the annual meeting of the American Diabetes Association, San Francisco Bay Area–based Tethys BioSciences announced
its development of a new test for Type 2 diabetes. The test was based
on a previous research cohort of nearly seven thousand individuals in
a population-based primary prevention study of cardiovascular disease in Denmark. Distinguished as a test of Type 2 diabetes risk, the
PreDx™ Diabetes Risk Score (DRS) claims to predict one's chances of
developing Type 2 diabetes within five years. In other words, the test
offered an opportunity to predict the onset of pathological sweetness
before the body does, and in so doing highlighted contrasting medical,
social, and market definitions of risk, diagnosis, and prognosis.

The ambiguous definitional tension between and social interpretation of diagnosis and risk prediction is all the more amplified by
the name PreDx: *Dx* is medical shorthand for *diagnosis*. So, does the
PreDx™ *predict*? Or, is it a *prediagnosis*? Is *prediagnosis* the same as *early
diagnosis*? As we will explore, the answers to these questions fall short
of clarifying whether early diagnosis constitutes prediction or diagnosis itself.

Just a year before, in May 2008, Tethys preceded its American Diabetes Association (ADA) presentation with an announcement launching the DRS in the local press. Ironically, the *San Francisco Chronicle*
called the DRS a "risk test" in the article title, but a "diagnostic test"
within the piece itself.[1] What makes the PreDx™ DRS innovative lies
in its claims to a predictive accuracy 50 percent greater than the most

reliable current Type 2 diabetes diagnostic test—the oral glucose tolerance test (OGTT). But unlike earlier diabetes risk scores, the PreDx™ DRS has an invasive component: a blood draw is required to measure both serum cholesterol and triglyceride levels. The PreDx™ DRS is not an innovative technology in the form of new hardware but rather a risk calculation engine based on physiological biomarkers and familial assessments in a preidentified population of high-risk individuals.

In collapsing diagnostic and predictive temporal frames, the DRS exemplifies new discursive and interpretive possibilities: a technology that further redefines risk as diagnosis in reordering narratives about the structure of the natural, social, and, I suggest, economic worlds.[2] In this chapter, I seek to show how "technological artistry" masked the attempted recruitment and subsequent translation of African American risk into universal Type 2 risk for broader clinical and market acceptance of the Tethys Diabetes Risk Score.[3] I offer a case where categorical thinking presumed, in error, that race *performs* predictably as biology.

PREDICTING PATHOLOGICAL SWEETNESS

Diabetes risk scores were first developed around the turn of the century to identify individuals with a high probability of developing Type 2 diabetes.[4] Using regression analyses, diabetes risk calculations offered the possibility of noninvasive screenings of large population groups while also avoiding expensive and time-consuming laboratory tests.[5] Moreover, the development of diabetes risk score algorithms sought to address the need for cost-effective public health screening among the uninsured, not as a profit-producing marketable commodity covered by private insurance. Early diabetes risk scores originated in Denmark and Finland among putatively homogeneous populations. For this reason, the originators of the Finnish Diabetes Risk Score, the DETECT-2, in citing the homogeneity of its research population as a methodological weakness, expanded its study to Mauritius, a predominantly Afro-Creole and South Asian island nation in the Indian Ocean, to obtain the heterogeneous, high-risk population sample that researchers desired.[6]

Important to this discussion, the question of precisely when the link between race and diabetes risk actually occurred remains unknown.[7] I suggest that the answer depends on the biopolitical agendas specific to certain nation-states. Different ethnic groups inhabit different levels of risk in different national diabetes risk scores. For example, the Australian Diabetes Risk Score assigns high risk to "Aborigines, Torres Strait Islanders, Maoris and Pacific Islanders."[8] On the UK Diabetes risk-score website, the individuals shown and made narratively available at the click of a mouse were overwhelmingly South Asian. The site features neither Afro-Caribbeans nor Africans visually, nor does it refer to these groups textually.[9]

To this point, the American Diabetes Association Diabetes Risk Test does not include race as a calculable variable. However, the bottom of the test form mentions that those of African American, Native American, Hispanic/Latino, and Asian/Pacific Islander ancestry tend toward higher Type 2 diabetes risk. Therefore, while not included in the test, race and ethnicity remained an independent variable of inestimable significance in an ostensibly race-neutral assessment. These examples highlight the variable estimations of race and diabetes risk in the sovereign biopolitics of different national formations.

Today, dozens of diabetes risk scores exist around the world. Some risk scores exemplify unique demographic characteristics of bounded nation-states (e.g., Australian, Chinese, Indian, German, American, Finnish, UK, Danish, etc.) or the private sector, such as the PreDx™ Diabetes Risk Score. Clinical as well as university (i.e., Framingham, Cambridge) research institutions have also developed diabetes risk-prediction models, some amalgams of the PreDx™ DRS and older diagnostic technologies such as the OGTT or the hemoglobin A1C test.[10] The primary difference between the nation-state's diabetes risk score and the biomarket risk score of the private sector rests in the applied reach of the technology that each envisions. Although national and institutional diabetes risk scores have ready applicability in their respective clinical spheres, private-sector risk scores such as the Tethys DRS seek to occupy not only these older biopolitical clinical spaces but also the biocapital circuits of the international diabetes market; the PreDx™ DRS does not include race as a risk-assessment category, using "family history" instead.[11]

My concern links the development of diabetes risk-prediction technology with my previous examination of the medicalization of "prediabetes" and whether that risk should be addressed through pharmaceutical approaches. I show next how risk, race, and speculation figured in the development of the PreDx™ DRS, revealing a market approach based on the idea that asymptomatic people, whom Charis Thompson calls "pre-vivors," have predictable medical futures that can, and should, be medicalized before they appear.[12]

THE BIOETHICS OF RACIAL RECRUITMENT

I contacted Betty Washington in the spring of 2009 about conducting participant observation and interviews at the diabetes prevention program she runs at the Alameda County Department of Public Health. Herself a Type 2 diabetes patient, she made it clear that if not for her employer-provided medical coverage, she would be uninsurable.[13] "A diabetes diagnosis marks people," she said. After discussing my project, she provided support in terms of interviews and introduced me to several of her staff of certified diabetes educators, one of whom, Darlene, I shadowed in the field. The diabetes program is housed within a maze of offices in what was once a former shopping center in East Oakland. Betty's diabetes educators teach classes in English, Spanish, Chinese, Hindi/Urdu, and Vietnamese, among other languages.

According to Betty, a local biotechnology company, Tethys Bio-Sciences, the creator of the PreDx™ Diabetes Risk Score, attempted to implement DRS testing locally between two groups of African Americans: junior-high-school-aged children and adult prediabetics. In the case of the children, they proposed testing in schools to determine the number of at-risk individuals present in a high-Type 2-risk youth population. Over two hundred thousand people under the age of twenty have been diagnosed with either Type 1 or Type 2 diabetes (estimates of undiagnosed diabetes are not available for this youth population).[14] This brought into ethical tension the opportunity to both test the DRS instrument and gain a clearer understanding of the numbers of latent diabetics existing within specific high-risk age groupings.

Betty related that in light of ethical issues surrounding consent, Tethys decided against pushing for DRS testing of school-age children in favor of testing adult prediabetics. She said that, nevertheless, "Tethys really wants to test its DRS on a large group of African Americans. They want to test their instrument on a high-risk Type 2 diabetes population and produce data that will confirm the effectiveness of the risk score. Presenting evidence based on a relatively homogeneous Danish population is not convincing enough." Though Tethys

BioSciences sought to recruit an African American sample population to test their new DRS technology, the risk calculation that the company's technology produces does not employ racial categories as an assessment variable. Innovation therefore depended on successfully subsuming the racial categories of the nation-state, in this case African Americans, into the technology, within contemporary neoliberal market forces of globalized Type 2 diabetes risk.

For example, scholars have shown that supposedly homogeneous populations have been constructed as such as part of various nationalist projects, for which Denmark is no exception.[15] In the United States, however, the strategy has never been to present the nation as racially homogeneous. Historically, biomedical research in the United States has proceeded with various adaptations to and co-optations with a racialized American polity.[16] One of the results following increasing demands for inclusion in biomedical research has been the rise in niche biomedical markets indexed to racialized groups.[17] This has fostered new approaches for recruiting and enrolling at-risk populations in bioscientific research that Steven Epstein termed "recruitmentology."[18] Moreover, technological innovation continues alongside older narratives linking illness risk with notions of race.[19] Over the last decade, these technological innovations and resurgent discussions about race and risk have occurred during a robust period of pharmaceutical company expansion.[20] Although Betty Washington's diabetes educators work with a diverse set of high-risk populations representing larger potential sample sizes, for reasons perhaps to do with population, location, and relative residential segregation, none of these groups were as desirable for recruitment as African Americans in Oakland.

The proponents of the PreDx™ DRS cited its cost savings over the lifetime of a Type 2 diabetes patient due to the test's early-warning capability.[21] Betty saw this cost-saving claim as part of both the assumption and market justification driving Tethys's effort to test African American prediabetics. The company's five-year risk prediction to Type 2 diabetes onset model, she explained, offered a motivational incentive to create more committed changes in diet, lifestyle, and pharmaceutical practices in the newly aware subject. While I cannot claim that Tethys saw African Americans as a *central* research population, they comprised, like those in Mauritius, a *desirable* research population for testing DRS technology. But to make the DRS truly marketable by gaining clinical acceptance and increasing venture capital infusions, Tethys could surely use those African American research participants to better calibrate the instrument. How to best recruit them?

RECRUITING BLACK RISK

Four months after interviewing Betty Washington, I walked through downtown Oakland to Jack London Square for the local annual American Diabetes Association Step Out! Walk Against Diabetes event. A woman named Minnie and I struck up a conversation as we headed to the event. She was recognizable in her red t-shirt as a Step Out! volunteer, and after I told her about my research, she said, "That's good. We all need to fight against this terrible disease. I know it will kill me one day. Everyone in my family has it. I know it's coming for me, too. I might even have it now, but I don't want to know. As you get older, your chances go way up, especially for a middle-aged Asian lady with my family history. We have to find a cure." Arriving at the event site, Minnie and I exchanged contact information, bade our respective farewells, and went on our separate ways. By coincidence, Minnie worked as an administrator for one of the two large drugstore chains in the area, CVS and Walgreens, which, along with Genentech, were secondary sponsors of the event. She later told me of CVS's recent acquisitions and mergers across the United States. "They plan to eventually operate around 100 pharmacies in San Francisco alone. Walgreens already has seventy-five stores in San Francisco," she said. That works out to around one CVS or Walgreens drugstore for every fifty residents of the city of San Francisco. "This is a battle for the Type 2 diabetic dollar," Minnie averred.[22] Her comments lent rationality to why both drugstore chains were present and cosponsoring the Step Out! Against Diabetes Walk.[23]

On the event stage, a DJ played music while doubling as the event's master of ceremonies. James Brown's "I Feel Good" set the thematic backdrop and tone for the event: "I feel nice, like sugar and spice." However, the discursive center of event attention was the main corporate sponsor, Tethys BioSciences, a fact the DJ mentioned at least every ten minutes, or two songs, over the course of an hour and fifteen minutes. With each announcement, he implored the crowd to make sure and visit the Tethys table, "where their representatives are eager and ready to talk to you."

Before the walk began, after a diagnosed Type 2 diabetic tearfully recalled her struggles with the illness, a Tethys vice-president took to the microphone. He reiterated the company's commitment to fighting diabetes, but immediately followed with, "There are over fifty-seven million prediabetics in the country, and what we want is to develop early-detection models that can get people involved earlier in diabetes prevention and treatment." He made no mention of existing diagnosed diabetics like the preceding speaker, undiagnosed or hidden diabetics, or anything concerning Type 2 diabetes itself. Marketing hat on, he decentered the theme of the day from diagnosed Type 2 diabetes to future Type 2 diabetes risk, which his company proffered to predict. In making a temporal shift from diagnosis to risk prediction, he medicalized diabetic risk in terms of either prevention or treatment.

I decided to visit the company's table and speak to their "eager and ready" representatives. I met the director of marketing development and another company vice-president, both of whom greeted me enthusiastically. Another employee, African American, constituted the third member of the Tethys booth. After I described my research, the vice-president stepped back rather abruptly, leaving the director of marketing development to explain the company's recruiting rationale. Meanwhile, the African American employee busied herself with other tasks. When I asked about the applicability of the Inter99 Danish cohort data to the diverse U.S. Type 2 diabetic epidemiological map, the director of marketing development informed me that this is precisely why Tethys was seeking to attract interest among high-risk African American populations.

And such were the best-laid plans. Although the African American population in the San Francisco Bay Area ranks second only to Los Angeles in the state of California, the diabetes walk garnered a low African American turnout. In fact, there were more African American volunteers than walkers, the majority health-professions students from local colleges. Moreover, the layout of the Jack London Square walking course consisted of a one-mile loop circled three times. After the first mile, fully one-half of the walkers abandoned the course and promptly availed themselves of the free lunches a regional supermarket chain had provided. At the end of the second mile, perhaps one-quarter of the original participants continued. As I completed the third mile, most walkers had already left the event. With photographs taken, friends and acquaintances reunited, and donations given, participants abandoned the site. I was the only person who approached the Tethys table before the walk began, and I saw no visitors to their table as I completed each loop of the course. By the end of the walk, they had already started breaking down the booth.

RECRUITMENT RATIONALES

Both the ADA and Tethys in particular seemed misinformed about the social rhythms and community contexts necessary to generate robust research-participation interest from African Americans. If it is assumed, as I discuss later, that churches are indispensable to enlisting African American participation in various biomedical efforts, then Sunday morning is not the best time to generate interest and participation from that targeted at-risk Type 2 population—James Brown notwithstanding. The situation brought to light the incommensurability produced when applied recruitmentology misses its intended public mark.

I was unable to find out how many people Tethys sought to attract or their target sample size. However, the director of marketing development's comments, along with the Oakland venue, made sense regarding which group composed the envisioned target population. As I noted above, developers of diabetes risk scores saw research limitations in employing data from predominantly Northern European populations, with the Finnish group eventually moving their project to Mauritius, a predominantly Afro-Creole and South Asian former French sugar colony in the Indian Ocean. Further, Betty Washington's comments, based on her evident knowledge of the Danish study and its perceived limitations, lent credence to the idea that Tethys imagined local African Americans to be a diverse biological resource. Moreover, Tethys staffed their booth with an African American employee at that event, less than four blocks from Chinatown.

Minnie, as related earlier, was more concerned about finding a cure for diabetes than early detection of the illness. But it appeared that in the absence of a Mandarin or Cantonese-speaking employee, her demographic was ignored in favor of an African American, who during the hour I sat outside the Tethys booth spoke neither language. Helping "middle-aged Asian ladies" like Minnie and her diabetes-ravaged family depended on an instrument further calibrated with increased precision, not by Asian Americans, but by recruited and technologically embedded African Americans. From James Brown to the bio-technology company and dual national-chain pharmacy sponsorship, at the Oakland Step Out! Against Diabetes Walk, "recruitmentology" as a form of applied knowledge and practice, enabled by venture capital and constrained by its own cultural specificity, appeared to have failed that day.

Yet, Tethys arguably established a rhetorical presence and further contributed to technoscientific narratives of risk. Situating risk narratives front and center of an imagined Type 2 future refocuses attention to biocapital not as speculation but as a noble driver of a research-and-development vehicle for medical justice. The mise-en-scène at Jack London Square brought to light the ways race, risk, and capital seek to articulate the discursive logic of promissory futures. Creating a persuasive narrative of risk formed part of larger translational effort at making race, risk, and the future fungible components of an innovative technology.

TRANSLATING IDEAS INTO INCOME

Declan Butler's 2008 article "Translational Research: Crossing the Valley of Death," describing the gap, or valley, between translational research and improved health outcomes, elicited an outpouring of responses from clinical scientists, venture capitalists, and biotechnology and pharmaceutical stakeholders.[24]

Butler argued:

> Over the past 30 or so years, the ecosystems of basic and clinical research have diverged. The pharmaceutical industry, which for many years was expected to carry discoveries across the divide, is now hard pushed to do so. The abyss left behind is sometimes labeled the "valley of death"—and neither basic researchers, busy with discoveries, nor physicians, busy with patients, are keen to venture there.[25]

Clinical and biotechnological translation has been defined in various ways: from bench to bedside, ideas to health outcomes, ideas to income, science into market value, and between academy and industry. During my earlier 2004 Silicon Valley medical technology research with the Institute for the Future as well as networking with physicists and engineers in the area from 1995 to 2004, I became acutely aware of these newer definitions of scientific translation as the term gained in currency. I had met faculty who not only collaborated with the private sector but also founded start-up technology companies and served on the boards of directors of others. Networks of faculty scientist-entrepreneurs extended beyond national borders, from China to Scotland to both Cambridges, and from Bangalore to Palo Alto.

Moreover, the overwhelming majority of these scientist-entrepreneurs were faculty at private universities such as Stanford, MIT, and Heriot-Watt University in Scotland. The relative absence of public university faculty intrigued me well into the period of this research project. As my previous experience had been with Stanford and Heriot-Watt faculty entrepreneurs and private industry researchers, concerns about the "corporatization" of the academy, while perhaps relevant, did not surface within these research communities, or at the time in the mind of this nascent researcher. As members of the Institute of Electrical and Electronics Engineers (IEEE) and the International Society for Optics and Photonics (SPIE), these applied scientists fostered relationships between the academy and industry that appeared almost seamless. This was a very different but not dissimilar planet to the technological worlds of pharma and biotech, that of optical engineers and applied physicists. I nonetheless breathed the same Silicon Valley air, as did pharma, biotech, and applied physicist-researchers—and I, too, declared it good. Toward the end of the first decade of the twenty-first century, the public research sector decided to enjoin more extensive relationships with biotechnology, pharmaceutical, and venture capital interests in bringing science to the market in delivering better health outcomes in patients.

In 2010, at a South San Francisco biotechnology and venture capital conference, I met an official from the University of California, San Francisco, Office of Technology Transfer. When I mentioned my previous experiences in Silicon Valley, Dr. Abrego admitted, "Public universities have been slow to participate in private industry collaborations. UCSF recognizes this and is committed to becoming a major player. That is why I'm here." To this end, in 2006 UCSF opened the Center for BioEntrepreneurship (CBE) on its new Mission Bay Campus. The center's charge to "educate and enable scientist interaction with the venture capitalist sector" consisted in part of classes taught by industry experts. Translation in this pedagogical context means guiding scientists through the process of transforming an idea into an initial public offering (IPO) on the market. The center provided a space where academic researchers could present innovative ideas and helped facilitate working teams of research and venture capital stakeholders in developing these ideas, writing a business plan, and pitching the completed business plan to potential investors.

GOING TO TRANSLATION CAMP

I was invited by UCSF to attend Camp Entrepreneur, an attempt to introduce the university research community to its Center of BioEntrepreneurship as well as its efforts at fostering ties between the public university and the private sector. In light of my previous Silicon Valley experiences and meeting Dr. Abrego, I wanted to see how these efforts were taking shape. Further, I was interested in better understanding venture capital and biotech perspectives about what exactly constitutes potential value and how academic researchers could come to inhabit the language of the market. Specifically, I wanted to get a clearer picture of the current market and research environment that Tethys BioSciences operated within as it attempted to translate its clinical science into income and market share.

Camp Entrepreneur was held in Genentech Hall on UCSF's Mission Bay Campus.[26] An arguably appropriate venue, as Genentech was cofounded by UCSF research scientist Herbert Boyer in the late 1970s.[27] While Boyer was based in a public university, the fact that Genentech began with private venture capital funding illustrates, in selective retrospection, the possibilities of venture capital (or shall I say, biocapital) in contrast with the constraints of traditionally more conservative merchant bank capital. The die had been cast.

A large multinational bank interested in fostering deeper relationships between the academy and industry sponsored the camp. The meeting was opened by Maninder Kahlon, a neuroscientist with experience founding start-up tech companies in Silicon Valley, and who then served as the chief information officer of the Clinical and Translational Science Institute (CTSI) in the UCSF School of Medicine. "Let me see a show of hands. How many of you are MDs?" A smattering of hands went up. "OK, I'll say 25 percent. How many of you are PhDs— wow, 60 percent. Now, how many of you are in the venture capital or industry sector? I'll say 15 percent?"

Kahlon opened the floor to introductions by audience members asking what brought them to Camp Entrepreneur, what questions they had coming in, and what they hoped to take out of the experience. A venture capitalist introduced himself as having contributed to several start-up companies, with the overall experience having left him "frustrated":

> For me it's a question of translating science into market value—how to move translational science from the Office of Technology Transfer to the private sector? And what are the secrets and keys to making the shift from academic science to the market possible?

Another venture capital stakeholder followed, impatient with the entire translational pipeline from basic research to product development:

> The academic sphere is too slow in getting its research out, and biotech and pharma are incredibly wasteful with R and D [research and development] money. When it comes to innovation and market value, from what I've seen, corporate strategies see creating repeat users as more lucrative and important than creating new product.

Kahlon agreed that new therapeutic interventions have not kept pace with the amount of scientific research and funding channeled toward these innovative projects:

> The NIH [National Institutes of Health] responded by establishing the Center for Translational Science Awards [CTSA]. In 2006, UCSF received a five-year, $117 million award for the creation of the Center for Translational Science Institute [CTSI] here at UCSF. UCSF and Harvard are the largest recipients of this funding. Our mission is to accelerate research to bring health to more people more quickly.

At the time, the amount of funding NIH provided for translational research amounted to around 1 percent of its total research budget. The majority of funding was allocated to basic research. Despite these outlays, both public and private sector research did not produce the medical breakthroughs justified by the amounts of funding spent over the twenty-year period before 2010. For example, the FDA reported that in 2008, almost 800,000 biomedical research papers were published, but only two new drugs were approved by the agency.[28]

In an effort to revitalize scientific discovery, the CTSI aimed to facilitate matchmaking between science and industry as well as between successful scientists and CTSI staff, many if not most of whom, like Kahlon, have significant experience in the high-tech and venture capital sectors. She contrasted the "Old World" with the "New World" model the CTSI represents:

> Old World model scientists used to entertain private sector interest in their work usually through individual efforts—Internet searches and seeking and securing valuable mentorship which could provide an entrée into private sector venture capital networks. The New World model that the CTSI hopes to create centers on creating a one-stop site containing all potential sites of intramural funding and venture capital collaboration. We help researchers demonstrate measurable research changes in community health at the end of the translation chain.

As part of introducing academic researchers to the ethos and praxis of the market, UCSF, through the CTSI, now charges researchers a fee for these services after the first hour of consultation. "We don't want to turn good scientists into bad entrepreneurs. We can't force them to become entrepreneurs, but we know that there are good scientists out there who would make great entrepreneurs. We just have to find them and provide resources necessary to facilitate their work and nurture their entrepreneurial spirit."

I wondered how exactly a nurtured entrepreneurial spirit could help animate the good scientist's conceptualization of and approach to robust research. However, this comment describes the zeitgeist of scientific practice, where science and entrepreneurship exist dialectically in the production of new knowledges, technologies, and forms of health. The waste of both private and public research funding in the past and poor health outcomes hollowing the present valley of death now demands labor from the science of the biopolitical nation-state, or the public research sector. The ascendant but conditional biocapital formation outlined by Sunder Rajan today inversely desires to make biopolitics work for it. Crudely put, public sector science must no longer "see like a (nation-)state," it must "see like the (global) market," and reorient research accordingly.[29]

The inherent ambiguities of anticipating profit through calculated illness risk embraces the economic rationale of the biomedical market, of which the DRS, for example, is a part. But as discussed in the previous chapter, it also embraces, if not requires, the predictive and diagnostic ambiguities inherent to these technologies and interpretive frameworks. Assuming present risk based on recent basic research makes these innovative biotech and biopharma futures possible. Risk and research continue to find greater logical synchronicity in both public and private laboratories and clinics. In the case of diabetes, evaluating risk takes on different research imperatives and forms of inclusion within public biopolitical and private biocapital (or biomarket) spheres.

MARKET BODIES, MARKET POTENTIALS

Unlike glucometer technology or pharmaceuticals, whose marketing plans envision growing consumer bases of repeat buyers, a diabetic risk-score assessment is a one-time-use technology.[30] Therefore, from a global perspective, it is questionable whether idealized forms of medical inclusion in the United States could garner the market share promised by the changing demographic, economic, and epidemiological factors driving the Type 2 diabetes epidemic/pandemic. China's economic rise and the subsequent increase in its urban population, combined with its previous one-child policy, have facilitated a doubling of its Type 2 diabetic population in the last twelve years to nearly fifty-seven million individuals—a number nearly equal to the entire population of the United Kingdom, and more than double the entire U.S. Type 2 diabetic population. Added to this phenomenon, the Chinese health care system has been quickly moving toward a single-payer model. The emergence of this large and exponentially expanding population of Type 2 diabetes patients/consumers—in an economically prosperous society with sufficient resources to pay for out-of-pocket medical expenses—portends a boom in the Type 2 diabetes market.[31] Given the growing number of confirmed Type 2 diabetes cases in China, one can extrapolate the number of hidden or undiagnosed diabetics and prediabetics in the country. Of particular significance is the number of individuals in China who currently are at risk of developing Type 2 diabetes. It then becomes possible to imagine the potential of the PreDx™ DRS market in China alone.

Further, India, the nation with the largest number of Type 2 diabetics in the world, is experiencing smaller, albeit geometrically significant, rises in Type 2 diabetes as it, too, becomes increasingly prosperous economically.[32] Therefore, I ask whether medical inclusion regarding predictive and diagnostic instruments such as the PreDx™ DRS in the United States are economically relevant, necessary, or even anticipated marketing drivers of Type 2 diabetes technological research and deployment. Perhaps even more significantly, class crosscuts both China and India's Type 2 diabetes populations in ways inverse to the U.S. phenomenon. While obesity and Type 2 diabetes in the United States disproportionally affect lower socioeconomic groups and have penetrated deep into rural areas of China and India, the increase in Type 2 diabetes since the turn of the century corresponds to both countries' rising urbanized middle and upper classes.[33] These demographic and socioeconomic factors make both nations attractive long-term prospects for future diabetes-industry efforts at market penetration. Although market logic on this side of the Atlantic and Pacific sees China and India as future sites of U.S. biotechnological penetration, several problems trouble any robust short-term success.

At the 2010 gathering of venture capital executives and clinical and biotechnology researchers in South San Francisco mentioned earlier, I came to better understand the contemporary urgency of biotechnological profitability within the then current economic and regulatory zeitgeist of biocapital. Conducted by a private biotechnology and venture capital consortium in the San Francisco Bay Area, the meeting's organizers brought together those seeking funding with the funders themselves. Before the meeting, research scientists looking for start-up or next-stage funding circulated around the room, making pitches and proposals of arranged marriage to the venture capitalists. My focus centered on the economic and regulatory climate for U.S. biotechnology firms seeking to enter Chinese and Indian Type 2 diabetes markets. I struck up a conversation with a Silicon Valley venture capital partner about the situation.

Ronald made it clear that U.S. biotechnology and pharmaceutical firms desiring entry into the Chinese, Indian, and even European health care markets face many hurdles:

The United States remains the best return on investment [ROI] dollar health care investor nation in the world. There are too many rules and regulations in the various European countries. European penetration requires strong distribution links that are difficult to forge. Yes, China and India's Type 2 diabetes populations and increasing wealth appear, on surface, lucrative sites for future investment. However, they should both be viewed within long- rather than short-term investment strategies: China is a regula- tory nightmare; in India, medical devices find distribution mainly through physician networks. Therefore, both present distinct but powerful distribution problems. One needs a global partner to penetrate either market.

Ronald added, "Despite its growing economy, India has not yet devel- oped a consumer base sufficient to meet the demands and expecta- tions of international capital investors in biomedical technology and pharmaceutical firms." But while the challenges facing Western market penetration into the subcontinent preclude any short-term financial reward, it remains a vast repository of biovalue for Type 2 diabetes re- searchers. According to Ronald, "India has the largest number of cases of diabetic nephropathy [kidney disease] among Type 2 diabetics in the world. This makes it a great place to conduct offshore clinical trials. There are CROs [private clinical research organizations] everywhere and the FDA accepts research conducted by these CROs among In- dian populations."

Despite India's large pool of Type 2 diabetics, they pose a classi- ficatory problem: How to classify subcontinental populations ethni- cally and racially? Nineteenth-century European racial demarcations between "Aryan" North India and "Dravidian" South India offered narrative affirmation of Western dominance over darker Others in the rest of the world.[34] Subsequent efforts by the British to equate caste with race resulted in over two thousand "castes" not only de- fined in their original terms, namely, by occupation, but expanded to conflate occupation with behavior as an inherited form of pheno- typical expression.[35] North/South and caste/behavior became ra- cialized voluminously in ways that still influence political, social, and scientific attention in India today. In the absence of a coherent cat- egorical box driving a categorical imperative that both rationalizes and motivates research that would reliably generate convincing data,

African-descent populations serve a classificatory purpose not yet fully demarcated in India.[36]

In the midst of these ambiguous classificatory and bioeconomic realities, critiques of the PreDx™ Diabetes Risk Score began to mount after its introduction. In the ensuing debate, both race and ethnicity came under closer scrutiny, with their relevance to the diabetes risk-prediction algorithm calibration questioned qualitatively by other researchers, eventually by Tethys, and later, fatally, by the market.

PUSHING BACK ON FUTURE CLAIMS

From its introduction, Tethys faced clinical pushback concerning the PreDx™ Diabetes Risk Score, its biostatistical methodologies, and claims of superior predictive power. In 2010, a group of German researchers contended that the Tethys model would produce false-positive results of upwards of 40 percent. These researchers saw the Framingham, Cambridge, and German risk models as statistically superior:

> Analyses of the power of biomarkers to identify high-risk individuals are worthwhile. However, measurement of some of the suggested biomarkers is costly, and therefore, efforts toward a careful comparison and appraisal of different methods to predict diabetes risk have to be made. Also, diabetes risk screening is still hampered by a large number of false-positive screening results at acceptable sensitivities and consequently by large numbers needed to treat with lifestyle interventions. Thus, new prediction models should aim to optimize discrimination rather than to replace existing models.[37]

The German researchers doubted that a risk assessment that does not take smoking status, sex, and hypertension into account could in any way prove superior to existing models.[38] Moreover, unlike the authors of the DRS literature, the German scientists had no professional conflict of interest or affiliation with any commercial concern. In contrast, the original 2009 Tethys paper was coauthored between Tethys scientists and shareholders, and the 2010 response to Rathmann, Kowall, and Schulze written solely by Tethys scientists and Inter99 Danish researchers. Rathmann, Kowall, and Schulze suggested that the DRS model is no better than simple clinical models and thus is of limited utility.

To support this contention, they compare our area under the receiver operating characteristic curve (AROC) with those reported for different models. However, the AROC of a test is population specific; therefore, comparisons between populations with different baseline risks are problematic because sensitivity and specificity are subject to alteration by disease prevalence.[39]

The Tethys authors argued that while the evaluative standard employed by Rathmann, Kowall, and Schulze was population specific, comparative analyses between populations were problematic. Their response to the German group was that diet and lifestyle criteria from the Danish Inter99 cohort were "unavailable," and that sex, smoking, and hypertension did not "improve the performance" of the DRS. As such, they maintained that their DRS technology should not be compared with the German DRS. The authors cited data from the Inter99 Danish cohort to claim greater accuracy than other clinical risk scores, while emphasizing an improvement over questionnaire and algorithmic indexes of diabetes risk. This, despite the limited population sample the Danish cohort represents.[40] The larger sociobehavioral, environmental, and community factors potentially shaping epigenetic Type 2 diabetes prevalence and causation were elided in favor of biological markers of risk attributed to different subpopulations. In effect, Tethys researchers imagined different populations with different Type 2 diabetes baseline risk profiles offering more predictive power than sex, smoking, or hypertensive status. Without any specific mention of race, the responding authors' statement implied biological differences between groups, which DRS technology endeavors to delineate. In this way, risk and subpopulation both became relinked and rebiologized in terms of disease prevalence.

Tethys BioSciences eventually found a way to obtain an ethnically diverse and arguably disciplined research-subject pool. In May 2011, the company announced an agreement with the U.S. Air Force to test the PreDx™ Diabetes Risk Score and evaluate post-test motivation on select groups of former service personnel and their dependents.[41] This provided Tethys with access to a significant number of test subjects, including those of African descent, for whom less stringent human subjects and informed-consent protocols exist than for research among civilian populations, and less open to ethical scrutiny than conducting offshore trials. The solution repeated the oft-seen pattern of private biomarket interests building upon older state formations and institutions.

There was much at stake in these debates, biocapital sponsorships, and performances. The primary stake involved growing the asset value of the company, not the singular profitability of a commoditized item of exchange. Birch and Tyfield emphasize the need to consider contemporary forms of asset accumulation as distinct from older commodity-production models of generating value. Increased asset value of a company, as *a form of property,* drives demand for a commodity, whereas decreased exchange value, as a disaggregated *item of exchange,* slows demand for it.[42] Tethys's attempts at recruiting African American participation existed within wider efforts between 2008 and 2011 to cogently articulate the value of the PreDx™ DRS to clinicians, researchers, and the venture capital market. This attempted generation of value during a particularly risk-averse speculative moment highlighted the contingencies, constraints, and opportunities for building promissory asset value and avoiding relegation to commodity-value status. With pressure mounting on multiple fronts, Tethys found itself engaged in a frantic race against a fast-ticking venture capital clock.

GENERATING VALUE

The local African American recruitment effort was part of a larger global boom in Type 2 diabetes prevalence and the subsequently expanding diabetes market. As one flock of canaries in this particular speculative Type 2 diabetes goldmine, African Americans embodied research imaginaries of difference that subsumed and marked national, ethnic, and racial notions of diabetes risk susceptibility. The performative challenge for Tethys consisted of making persuasive claims about the future predicated upon an understanding of the biological past, a future that links the DRS's five-year predictive prognosis/diagnosis with speculation, and risk, both diabetic and market, with value.

But the company's timing could not have been worse. The unveiling of the Tethys PreDx™ Diabetes Risk Score in May 2008 came in the second year of a four-year decline in the venture capital investment model for funding biotechnology firms. Single investor "All-In" investments fell from a high of 87 percent in 2007 to 24 percent in 2011, as more conservative syndicate-partnered "structured" investments rose from 13 percent in 2007 to 76 percent in 2011. However, the most active period of venture capital investment restructuring occurred between 2007 and 2009, when single-investor funding dropped from 87 percent to 15 percent; while inversely, syndicate group funding grew from 13 percent to 85 percent.[43] It was in this risk-averse speculative moment that Tethys BioSciences unveiled the DRS.

As a general partner in a Silicon Valley venture capital company explained to me in 2010,

> 2009 was the worst year for biotechnology companies during this recession. These biotech companies currently worry over not only the commitment but also the viability of funding syndicates and networks into the near future. Health care technology financing dried up during the Internet and dot-com bubble during the mid to late 1990s. After the bubble burst in 1999, financing became scarce for both health care and Internet technology markets. . . . But 2009 was much worse.

He linked the events of the late 1990s and 2009 to the dyspepsia affecting venture capitalists' appetite for risk. "If today you tell a venture capital firm that your product will need a seven-year period from development to market entry—your presentation is over." Under such market conditions, a shorter window of time existed between generating a convincing increase in the asset value of an entire company and avoiding market relegation to commodity-value status as merely tangible, disaggregated items of exchange.

Risk-averse venture capital partnerships condition both the market opportunities and constraints that the contemporary diabetes pandemic/epidemic presents. The economic situation faced by biotechnology companies such as Tethys during the first decade of the twenty-first century demanded skillful negotiation through the rough currents of the venture capital market. This meant generating convincing data that would garner robust clinical acceptance in attracting greater market interest and adhesiveness. Toward achieving these clinical and market goals, African Americans were seen as a desirable research component of a racialized strategy to improve the predictive power of the instrument. Yet by 2012, Tethys had concluded that a company study of a *multiethnic* cohort found no significant risk predictability for Type 2 diabetes attributable to ethnicity, race, or gender.[44] Moreover, the German researchers were not alone in questioning the viability of the PreDx™ DRS for gaining clinical acceptance, not only as a predictive instrument, but also as a prescriptive tool.

I interviewed a leading clinical diabetes researcher and physician at a large public hospital in San Francisco who works with primarily low-income and minority patients, who noted,

> I would have to ask them, "Show me the money, I mean, show me the damn money! How will your risk score save me and my patients money and improve their health outcomes? How will your risk score help to arrest the progression of the disease in those with no health insurance, in poverty, and living on the environmental edge of health?" As it stands under these conditions, I struggle to help keep my patients' hemoglobin A1C levels under 8.0; even though we know that the desired level rests at 7.0 and below. But hell, to be honest, I'd be happy if all my patients were at 8.0. That's the reality of the situation, from my experience.

The market also remained unconvinced, and to a fatal degree. As of 2013 Tethys BioSciences was one of several diagnostics companies having sourced over $100 million in venture capital funding. Under these overexposed conditions, a positive financial exit for investors now depended on the successful commercialization of the companies' products, not the marketization of its stock.[45] Ultimately, Tethys's attempt to calibrate racial risk into its DRS technology failed its own clinical test, and in building company asset value, failed the market test as well: By the end of 2013, Tethys BioSciences was no longer in business.[46] The interpretive lenses through which risk-prediction technologies such as the DRS failed to reckon human difference complicated their strategies to clearly articulate their value—both to clinicians and investors. The case of the Tethys Diabetes Risk Score illuminates Althusser's term *overdetermination*. Tethys's recruitment effort at Jack London Square exemplified how the life sciences and technology are structurally and contextually overdetermined by the dictates of diverse bioeconomic interests that seek to market, patent, and commodify life forms and processes.[47]

Protodiabetes as a physiological *descriptor* had given way to prediabetes as a diagnostic *marker*, creating productive ambiguity that ran along a discursive continuum from prevention to treatment. The definitional ambiguity of prediabetes justified a pharmaceuticalization of diabetes prevention in the present, whether or not progression to the full condition of pathological sweetness had occurred. Within this discursive and clinical opening, the diabetes risk score emerged as a numerical index of treatability. But the discursive and clinical openings did not translate into a successful market outcome. What Jutel and Nettleton allude to as a "social technology of diagnosis" explicates why the DRS presents a case of "breathing race into the machine" as in Braun's important work on the development of the spirometer.[48] It chronicles an attempt to *render race invisible within the algorithm* for global market applicability beyond the narrow biopolitical limitations of ethnic and racial attributions of risk within individual nation-states.

RACE, RISK, AND THE VALLEY OF DEATH

Tethys's desire to test an African-descent cohort reflected a growing trend to medicalize what is in fact a poorly defined condition. *Prediabetes* is a contested term with a contested history of boundary making and shifting prescriptive rationales ranging lucratively from prevention to treatment. The American Diabetes Association's rather opaque position on prediabetes as a physiological descriptor provided an interpretive framework for introducing pharmaceutical interventions for the "illness" that blurred the therapeutic lines between prevention and treatment. In becoming integral to Tethys's DRS, which in turn sought to link prediabetes to high-ticket pharmaceutical interventions and national-chain pharmacy expansion, race and risk came to justify pharmaceuticalization in this arena. One crucial market limitation to the Tethys DRS achieving robust, global profitability lay in the fact that diabetes risk-score technologies function as an assessment of asymptomatic people in the ambient population, and thus rarely include repeat buyers, unlike glucometer and insulin-delivery systems, whose strategic marketing plans aim at growing consumer bases of lifetime repeat buyers.

The case of the Tethys DRS tells a story of how structural articulations of racial categories of risk and market speculation intersected with and indexed discursive, institutional, and epistemic notions of knowledge value. However, value first had to be negotiated through a series of translational performances that, as anthropologist Anna Tsing has put it, occurred "in the limelight of those historical moments when capital seeks creativity rather than stable reproduction."[49] I link creativity-seeking capital to the notion of *race* in the generation of asset value to show that where science and technology are globalizing, as well as where they are failing to globalize, racialization plays a contingent role in the differentiation of both epistemic pathways and of markets.[50] Consequently, the case of the DRS exemplified an attempted alchemical transformation of race from an intangible asset into a tangible commodity, a new biotechnology coproduced from the raw material of social norms and status hierarchies.

The Valley of Death represents an all-too-real social space between the scientific community, the market, and patients, where the prematurely dead are buried in the absence of biotechnological deliverables. From within the valley floor, start-up companies sprouted by seed money planted deeply within the newly transported and terraced soil of basic science bloom fragrant flowers that will eventually bear the fruits of knowledge, health, and wealth. Where once there was death, there is life. Prognosis as predicate to speculation, because where there is hope there should be profit. Profit is health. Health is wealth. But nowhere in this narrative can we find a definition of translation as communicating and, most importantly, delivering science to the public from within a bioethical framework anchored firmly in the morass of the valley floor itself.

But as this chapter demonstrated and the next will relate, from the standpoint of cultural competence, understanding the racial metabolism of African-descent American communities remains a significant yet elusive research priority. Outreach to African-descent communities, as an integral part of organized recruitment, education, and data collection programs, continues to grapple with historical issues of trust. Clearly defining such an imagined community, and just who understands it best, blurs notions of *expert* and *expertise*—while, most importantly, illuminating the people and places where such knowledge might be found.

4

A Dark Past in Present Light

THE BLACK CHURCH, MEDICINE, AND TRUST

> I don't come to worry your patience.
> I just come to bring salvation.
> How do you do, everybody, how do you do?
>
> —"How Do You Do, Ev'rybody?" Greeting shout, from
> *The Long Road to Freedom: An Anthology of Black Music,*
> Harry Belafonte, compiler

As related, difficulties recruiting and subsuming race successfully as part of a larger biotechnological enterprise reflect a more persistent inability to understand the targeted population sociologically within their communities geographically. Over thirty years after the 1985 Report of the Secretary's Task Force on Black and Minority Health (also known as the Heckler Report), significant disparities in both health status and outcomes endure across ethnoracial groups. Yet, despite generating reams of empirical and quantitative data over the last three decades, the intersections of sociocultural, economic, community, and behavioral factors remain underexamined in health disparities research and underrepresented in policy.[1] In the relative absence of social, behavioral, and community-study research and policy impacts, these underutilized approaches have been recommended to better understand the social dynamics of communities and neighborhoods.[2]

Over a half century after the Framingham researchers implored for more strident attempts to conduct cardiometabolic research in relatively and strategically unknown geosocial communities, disparities, epidemiologists and, as we saw, biotechnology firms as research actors still seem unable to fully grasp the social rhythms resonant in African-descent groups. To the point of African-descent *groups,* this chapter argues for the definitional instability of a dynamic social group relegated to a static biopolitical category that exists amidst countervailing winds of a hegemonic blackness validated by history, power, and the nation. I aim here to shed greater light on the historical dynamism of the Negro, Black, and African American racial category in the United States. I expand its geographic raison d'être beyond national boundaries, to illustrate the challenges of recruiting African Americans for biomedical research with the offer of salvation while not worrying their patience.

But who is best positioned to dialogue and offer this promise? Who can do it without trying a patience well informed by history? The answers to these questions pivot between the community and the institution, each reflecting different epistemic orientations and approaches to reducing health disparities. In what follows, I suggest that diverse blackness decenters notions of "expert" and "expertise" in regard to the knowledge demands required and cultural skill sets acquired among community health workers (CHWs), certified diabetes educators (CDEs), and physician-researchers charged with fulfilling Framingham's promise.

THE BLACK CHURCH, MEDICINE, AND TRUST

Most scholarship examining health disparities among and cultural-competence efforts aimed at African Americans have tended to focus on community-based participation and other inclusionary paradigms.[3] However, little research has engaged the fundamental issue of trust and its intersections with the black church as a biomedical recruiting magnet stratified by gender, age, and class.[4] In this chapter, I connect a discussion of cultural competence and trust to the rise of the "health cabinet" or "health ministry" in predominantly African American churches over the last thirty years. Comprising health professional and lay members of church congregations, these outreach efforts emerged from within to address health and resource disparities in their respective communities and neighborhoods.[5]

In chapter 2, I mentioned that "the infected" African American would one day prove more valuable as a research subject than as a citizen deserving of timely and appropriate treatment. I bring that history forward with ethnographic work illustrating the ways memories of the unethical legacy of the Tuskegee Syphilis Study still loom large in the African American community. Given the long historical shadow of Tuskegee, questions persist about how to ethically recruit clinical research participants and conduct public health outreach to African Americans.[6] I explore the role of the black church as a venue for African American research recruitment and the limits to that approach. I suggest an inherent contradiction exists between the black church as an ethical site for establishing trust and biomedical recruitment in those spaces as an ethical undertaking. Further, I argue that class, educational, and cultural diversity within the putative black population complicate any singular understanding of both the black church and the African American racial category, and point to the need to reexamine the role of cultural competence in establishing overall professional competence. It is in these contested cultural and professional spaces this chapter interrogates trust as the fulcrum upon which successful inclusion efforts balance history, culture, and science.

I examine trust as a discursive index of "social robustness, the management and reporting of knowledge, and its underlying culture and systems of accountability."[7] Anthropological understandings of trust ethically demand more than a sociological understanding of dyadic relationships and forms of altruistic behavior. It requires a deeper engagement with history, power, and racialized affect. I present *community* here as an amorphous space where race, culture, risk, bodies, and history reproduce a social category of immense biovalue. I contrast that with *neighborhood* as an abstract template to circumscribe the ways communities are materially built, deconstructed, remade, and renamed as vectors for new forms of trust exchange. That is to say, changing neighborhood demographics highlight the ways unequal reserves of racial, cultural and social capital make different collective demands for its occupants, as in turn different demands are made upon them.[8] I answer anthropologist John Jackson's call in presenting not a black space, but a racialized space "blackened" by history, residential and economic segregation, and political and scientific classification. These "blackened" spaces reveal a demiworld of resource disparities irrespective of class status.[9] To be clear, in analyzing a community, I do not employ race as an analytical tool or instrument of accusation, but as a biopolitical category embedded within specific national histories indexing complex sets of social relationships, forms of exchange, and networks of trust.[10]

CATEGORICAL TRUST AND RACIAL RECRUITMENT

When I first contacted Dr. Asela in the summer of 2008 concerning my research, he warmly invited me to discuss both my project and the work of the Clinical Research Center (CRC).[11] Born and educated in Sri Lanka, he completed medical school in the United States and is one of a growing cadre of foreign-born or -trained endocrinologists practicing in the United States. Located in Rochester, New York, the CRC offers diabetes education classes for free to the public, from which it recruits volunteers for third-stage Type 2 diabetes clinical drug trials. As part of its clinical-trial recruitment, the center also conducts public education classes for patients suffering with hypertension, gout, and other metabolic disorders. The center's funding comes from pharmaceutical and biotechnology companies as well as public institutions like the National Institutes of Health.

I spent September and October 2008 attending the center's diabetes education class series. Dr. Asela, center staff, and a local physician took weekly turns lecturing on topics such as blood glucose monitoring, dietary practices, and physical activity, as well as addressing conditions associated with diabetes: hypertension, heart and kidney disease, and eye and foot problems. I conducted participant observation at these classes and formal and informal interviews with both Dr. Asela and several class attendees. During those six weeks, nearly sixty individuals attended these classes. Two African Americans attended in total, and of the two, the one who attended most did so for only the first two weeks.

After the first month, I asked Dr. Asela about the center's ability to perform successful outreach to the African American community. With frustration, he responded, "I have tried many approaches over time to try and attract more African Americans to our classes and workshops. I know about the history of Tuskegee and understand the reticence about participation in drug trials. I'm just trying to get them to come to the classes. I have come to the conclusion that I have to directly appeal to the [black] *churches* in order to create greater awareness about diabetes and interest in our work" (speaker's emphasis). As Dr. Asela referenced and another interlocutor will later mention, the Tuskegee Syphilis Study remains both a symbolic and cautionary narrative within the African American and biomedical community.[12] In the relative absence of trust, Dr. Asela found himself considering appealing to religious bodies of faith that represent a color-coded community with low social capital, embedded in a turbulent history of racialized bioevaluation and socioeconomic segregation.

Indeed, social scientific understandings of trust among targeted populations continue to occupy the strategic imaginations of various missionary (and biomedical) projects.[13] Building trust in biomedicine in the African American community after decades of well-placed distrust remains a challenge to those working in the areas of public health and health disparities research.[14] The black church has long served as an imagined venue where words could be trusted and social action sacralized.

The history of the African American church is one of a social movement organized along a continuum of passive accommodation, social control, and active social justice.[15] To this point, although many black churches developed health ministries and cabinets over the course of the twentieth century, most of these efforts crystallized as an outgrowth of the civil rights movement of the 1960s. The Black Panther movement organized health clinics as part of its political philosophy to equate medical justice with social justice.[16] Similarly, black physicians were at the forefront of the civil rights movement, often at their peril.[17] None of these efforts existed in political or cultural isolation from African American churches; often, they occurred with their tacit approval. In this way, I do not define the "black church" as a coherent monolithic or discursive entity but as a hierarchical social network reflecting a historically specific genealogy of collective aspirations rooted in a political economic language of social justice.[18]

Moreover, adding to Dr. Asela's frustration is the proximity of the CRC to Rochester's two largest predominantly African American communities: Southwest Rochester is less than a twenty-minute drive from the CRC, and Northeast Rochester is less than ten minutes away. While I was observing Dr. Asela and conducting research at the CRC, I was also doing parallel fieldwork in Southwest Rochester's African American community. Having spent a significant period of my life there, I knew many in the community living with Type 2 diabetes and associated conditions. From this multi-sited perspective and against the historical backdrop of trust, I examined one church's outreach efforts amid the diversity of the racial category *African American* in Rochester. However, in this diasporic and transnational *black* community, the postcolonial, postregime, and postblack subject is as embedded as the post–Jim Crow citizen—hence, my pointed use of the term *black* instead of *African American* church. I also highlight the gendered problematics of instrumentalizing religion to achieve robust outreach and recruitment goals within church spaces.

MT. ZION

Mr. and Mrs. Vitale called to invite me to a diabetes education workshop at their church in the center of Rochester's black community. "We would really like to see you there," Mr. Vitale said, "I think it would be good for you to see what is happening at the church and in the city with diabetes. It's terrible."

Mt. Zion Baptist Church reflects both the old and the new in a community steeped in the history of the abolition, women's rights, and civil rights movements. In 1996, congregants erected a new church building that beautifully enveloped the original 1906 structure in a separate wing. The church is located in the former Third Ward, one of two wards (out of twenty-four) in Rochester where African Americans were allowed to reside during socially enforced segregation until the early 1960s. Frederick Douglass lived and published the *North Star* in the Third Ward. Both the Susan B. Anthony House and the Frederick Douglass Museum straddle the Southwest Rochester and Maple Neighborhoods. After the abolition of slavery in New York State in 1827, the Memorial AME Zion Church became the first authorized, independent African American congregation in the city. Douglass first printed the *North Star* in the AME Church basement, less than a ten-minute walk from the future site of Mt. Zion Baptist Church.[19]

Despite this progressive history, residential and environmental constraints of de facto segregation in Rochester intensified with the growth of the African American community during the 1950s. Rochester's population had already reached its height in 1950.[20] At the beginning of that decade, around seventy-five hundred African Americans lived in the city. By 1959, the African American population had swelled to nearly fifty thousand individuals, mostly from the southern United States.[21] But as quickly as African Americans moved to the city, whites began moving out.

In July 1964, Rochester experienced rioting, which further accelerated white flight to the suburbs.[22] Earlier urban renewal and later

Great Society programs were accompanied by a slow hollowing out of the downtown area, which was all but gutted by the 1980s. Thereafter, the previously segregated Third Ward crossed the Genesee Street boundary that once separated it from the Nineteenth Ward to form the Southwest Rochester Neighborhood. The economic life of the city, including its supermarkets, migrated to the suburbs. Today, even the city's main post office is no longer located within the city itself. As of the 2010 census, Rochester's population has fallen 37 percent from its 1950 peak.[23] Essentially, the city has been subsumed within a larger countywide metropolitan area, leaving the Southwest Rochester Neighborhood ringed and bypassed by highways and expressways facilitating entry to the city center and exit to the surrounding suburbs.

Much of Mt. Zion's congregation, too, has dispersed outward from the Third Ward deeper into the former Nineteenth Ward and beyond into the surrounding suburbs. The church is located in a community and neighborhood devastated by the demise of the Eastman Kodak Company during the early 1980s, followed quickly on its heels by the crack cocaine epidemic of the 1980s and 1990s.[24] Urban planners and city managers, not only in Rochester but elsewhere, have decided that the best way to address crime and poverty is to build out and through these problems, dispersing the population outward from the center city.[25] Moreover, increasing gentrification during the last two decades has occurred in the Southwest Rochester Neighborhood, first in the Cornhill District bordering Mt. Zion and more recently near the University of Rochester. While gentrification unofficially aims to bring more whites back to the city, many African Americans, including much of Mt. Zion's congregation, have joined the exodus to the suburbs. Others have "return migrated" to the Southern United States, particularly Atlanta and North Carolina.[26] At the same time, an increase in immigrant African and Caribbean populations has somewhat counterbalanced the diminution of the city's older African American population.[27] Therefore, despite these intra- and international movements, Rochester's African-descent population arrived in the city relatively recently. Connections with Southern U.S. and transatlantic areas of origin remain robust, and in terms of the legacy U.S. African American population, a strong Southern cultural ethos persists.

Reverend Marlowe, Mt. Zion's interim pastor, explained the church's commitment to the community as we walked from the newer structure into the bosom of the older church. The "old" church, founded by the descendants of former slaves from a diverse range of states and regional cultures in the U.S. South, now houses a diverse congregation that includes members from the Caribbean and West Africa:

> We decided to build around the older church as a reminder of our beginning, where we came from and where we are going. It shows that our dedication to the community has not changed. Our new building holds firm to that original mission, but as a sign that the community itself is constantly changing. And our church, both the old and the new, reflects those changes and the importance of adapting to those changes. Our health work in the community is one part of this.

Reverend Marlowe spoke in even, measured tones. Magnanimous and managerial, he exemplified Du Bois's notion of the "Negro preacher" as someone more "executive" than "spiritual," both in demeanor and praxis.[28] Although he stressed the necessity of adapting to change, Reverend Marlowe was careful to emphasize the continuing social justice mission of Mt. Zion and its community health work. Although Mt. Zion has outgrown and enveloped its original building, it is neither a "megachurch" nor an ideological proponent of the "prosperity gospel." Megachurches are generally defined as congregations having two thousand or more members; Mt. Zion's congregation numbers less than fifteen hundred.[29] The church's historical role in the civil rights movement of the 1950s and 1960s remains at the forefront of its unwavering social justice mission in serving Rochester's African American community—a community more impoverished and undereducated now than it was twenty-five years ago.[30]

In response to health issues affecting the community and its members, Mt. Zion organized eleven health care teams. Each team serves as point persons for those living within a different zip code of the city. They help to arrange medical care and transportation for those in need as well as to generate interest in and volunteers for Mt. Zion's health programs, workshops, and fairs, such as its annual neighborhood reunion each August. Upon hearing of my research from a fellow church member, the Vitales, both retirees from the Eastman Kodak Company, invited me to Mt. Zion's Annual Diabetes and Alzheimer's Awareness Workshop.

TRUSTING A DARK PAST IN PRESENT LIGHT

Mt. Zion's diabetes education workshop was part of an incipient nationwide effort in 2008 by the American Diabetes Association to promote diabetes awareness and outreach through black churches. The ADA in cosponsorship with Rite Aid Pharmacy's new program, ID Day at Church (short for "I Decide to Stop Diabetes at Church"), signaled the beginning of activities marking American Diabetes Month in November. In concert with the National Baptist Convention, the program aimed to reach over 100,000 Americans on that day. The ID Day at Church effort sought to use the church as a venue to establish trust in communicating biomedical and public health messages about Type 2 diabetes to the high-risk yet historically distrustful African American community.[31] At the event, a former Rochester mayor and a local news anchor, both church members, gave keynote addresses concerning the gravity and spread of both Type 2 diabetes and Alzheimer's disease in the community. Another church member, Merlene Bailey, a community coordinator from the American Diabetes Association who presented on Type 2 diabetes self-care, would become my primary community contact. The assembled speakers focused their remarks on the effects of these illnesses on loved ones, the importance of increasing awareness in the community, and the perennial issue of trust in biomedical institutions.

In his statement to the audience, workshop leader Robert Mann said,

> I know why so many of you are here and not there at other
> diabetes education classes in the wider community. It's because
> you don't trust the message unless it comes from people who
> look like you [laughter and applause]. Since Tuskegee, we don't
> trust everything coming from medicine—and this won't be easily
> overcome. If you want to reach people of color, you have to have
> people of color in front of them.

As a methodological approach, Robert Mann's allusion to Tuskegee was not an argument in principle against biomedical interventions based on race and ethnicity. Linking medicine, race, and trust with history and their respective technoscientific assemblages, Mann argued for a phenotypically suitable representative of the intervention itself, what those in public health call "racial concordance."[32] The assumption that an African American biomedical practitioner or researcher would be trustworthy is, however, both questionable and problematic given the complicity of African Americans in the Tuskegee Syphilis Study itself.[33]

The Tuskegee Syphilis Study, a four-decade-long racial project examining the effects of untreated syphilis in African American men conducted from 1932 to 1972, revealed how fluent cultural competence can obfuscate rather than clarify bioethical questions of consent and inclusion. Moreover, as an ethical project, cultural competence did not cultivate trust based on access to timely and appropriate treatment. However, Tuskegee occurred in isolated areas of rural Alabama inhabited by relatively homogeneous African American demographic and cultural communities. Such is not the case with Rochester, where both post–Jim Crow and postcolonial black subjects have come to mutually occupy community and epidemiological space.

OF CULTURES AND COMPETENCE

The people constituting Rochester's African American community exemplify Glissant's assertion that political borders and nationalistic narratives obscure the fact that indeed "history travels with the seas," and for that matter in the contemporary, by air as well.[34] The policed borders of these narratives testify to a contested history of such journeys. The Immigration Act of 1965, which African American civil rights organizations did not support, opened immigration to the United States from the Caribbean, Africa, and Asia.[35] Successive waves from the Caribbean blended in and continually redefined Rochester's African American community, particularly from the former British West Indies, Puerto Rico, and post-Revolution Cuba. They are not necessarily a political community, but members of a shared, politically constructed, and economically stratified sociobiological category that obscures the politics both within and of the category, as well as their historical antecedents. Their journeys took them from agricultural to industrial revolutions, rural to urban spaces, colonial or Jim Crow subjecthood to national citizenship, and from majority to minority status, to the nodal point of Rochester.[36] As beneficiaries of that legislation, Merlene Bailey's mother migrated from Barbados and her father from Guyana; Merlene was born in Rochester.

In effect, Rochester's black community, like many today, comprises a combination and permutation of individuals, couples, families, and kinship networks extending to and from the Southern United States, the Caribbean, and Canada, to the United Kingdom, France, and Africa. More recently, immigrants from Africa, Haiti, Ethiopia, and the Dominican Republic have made the city home, along with an interstitial Arab shopkeeper class. Less than one block from Mt. Zion, the neighborhood Catholic parish priest is from Kenya, his predecessor from Trinidad, with a congregation consisting mainly of Louisiana Creoles, Nigerians, Trinidadians, Jamaicans, Puerto Ricans, Haitians, and Dominicans. Cities like Rochester expose normalizing and totalizing social, political, and racial hegemonies that discursively neglect the ongoing, qualitative redefinitions of biohistorical blackness in the United States, hegemonies that do not reflect the society at large. After all, most of the Caribbean is closer to Rochester than Rochester is to either San Francisco or Los Angeles.

Upon closer sociogenic examination, we find genealogies and ontologies of sugarcane, tobacco, cotton, rice, cacao, coffee, *khat,* and kola, metabolically linked within what anthropologist John Jackson calls a "blackened" categorical and community space. The cultural diversity and social dynamics of an ethnoracial category speaking in multiple registers and often different languages confound any static definition of a community and blur any singular historical optic for envisioning a comprehensive project toward such an imagined community.

In the case of Type 2 diabetes, public health and private biomedical interests continue to seek new ways of articulating information about the illness. If successful, the expertise gained could, inversely, prove useful for developing effective recruitment strategies for clinical research trials, Dr. Asela's dogged goal. Therefore, finding a common language attuned to rapidly changing communities imagined through ethnoracial lenses requires a cultural broker with an ear to the ground, one of considerable multicultural and often, multilingual competence. The struggle to competence involves two broad sets of actors, CHWs and CDEs. CHWs, seen as those with ears to the ground, and CDEs, seen as those with eyes on the science, challenge hierarchical notions of expert and expertise regarding the community. The individual, the clinic, and the community represent three different knowledge domains, as well as three different spatial imaginaries requiring broad competencies capable of garnering trust in each.

EXPERTISE IN THE ABSENCE OF EXPERTS

I situate this chapter within a discussion of expertise in the form and person of the endocrinologist and the pipeline issues affecting the shortage of physicians in the medical specialty. I begin this section with the epidemiology and future projections in the growth of Type 2 diabetes in the United States. I contrast this with the present shortage of endocrinologists and primary care physicians, which threatens the possible successful therapeutic futures of not only diabetes and the wider cardiometabolic syndrome, but the entire medical system as a whole. I suggest in this section that these shortages in professional labor further rationalize technological solutions and community interventions, necessarily shifting the burden of translational labor from the clinician to the community health worker.

Currently, one in three persons born in the United States today will develop Type 2 diabetes. One in six children in the United States are prediabetic; one in three obese children is prediabetic. One in two Latino Americans born today will develop Type 2 diabetes. According to the Centers for Disease Control (CDC) cases of Type 2 diabetes will triple by 2050, affecting one in every three adults in the nation.[37] Nevertheless, with nearly 26 million diagnosed and 6 million *hidden* or undiagnosed diabetics in the United States, fierce competition currently exists among manufacturers for domination of a burgeoning blood glucometer market growing by 1.6 million newly diagnosed Type 2 diabetics each year. Today, expenditures on diabetes comprise one out of every seven health care dollars.[38]

Further, it must be kept in mind that very few people die from diabetes. The majority of diabetics die from kidney failure or heart disease. Diabetics have a two-to-fourfold increased chance of dying from cardiovascular disease.[39] It is the microvascular complications and treatments arising from diabetes—permanent nerve damage, retinopathy, poor circulation resulting in limb amputations, decreased kidney functioning necessitating renal dialysis, pharmaceutical drugs, and so on—that drive the increasing cost of diabetes patient care. It is also worth noting that end-stage renal disease is the only universally covered illness in American medicine.[40] In other words, many diabetics do not become eligible for medical insurance until these life-threatening complications manifest themselves. This should give us pause to consider the economic, medical, ethical, and policy priorities and foci of the various institutions and interests terracing the topography of care of the U.S. diabetic medical landscape.

As of 2008, there was only one board-certified pediatric endocrinologist for every 17,000 obese children in the United States. Two states, Wyoming and Montana, had no board-certified pediatric endocrinologists. Massachusetts had the highest ratio of pediatric endocrinologists to obese children at roughly 1:5,000. Mississippi, the most obese state in the nation, had a ratio of nearly 1:100,000. According to Stewart,

> The endocrinologist shortage has impaired access to care by patients with diabetes, obesity, metabolic syndrome, lipid disorders, thyroid nodules, thyroid cancer, osteoporosis, pituitary disease, adrenal disease, menopausal symptoms, and reproductive disorders. It is standard to encounter waits of three to nine months and many endocrinology practices are closed to new patients.[41]

According to Darlene Pedraza from the Alameda County Department of Public Health, the three-county area of the East Bay of Northern California, with some of the wealthiest communities in the state, had only one board-certified endocrinologist in private practice in 2008. At that time, Santa Cruz County had only one board certified endocrinologist, located in North County, while the majority of the Latinx population resides in South County. In both California and New York, I was told by diabetes professionals of the lack of endocrinologists coming down the medical specialty chute. One physician and diabetes educator in San Francisco said that endocrinology isn't "sexy" to young medical students, who seek more lucrative careers in anesthesiology, cardiology, and surgical specialties, particularly cosmetic surgery.[42] Cardiologists in private practice are bringing in more endocrinologists to care for an increasing Type 2 diabetes patient load, which then allows cardiologists to concentrate on more economically lucrative medical practices.[43] While more foreign-trained endocrinologists are being recruited to fill in the gaps, their numbers are insufficient given the burgeoning Type 2 diabetes population.

An internist in San Francisco working with at-risk populations added to my professional pipeline question by posing another:

Yes, there is an endocrinologist shortage. Yes, there are those who believe that diabetics and the chronically obese should have access to endocrinologists. I wouldn't disagree with that, and I have had many discussions with my colleagues on this issue. But I always say [that] the real question is, "What is the best front-line medical specialty for addressing these problems, endocrinology or primary care?"

Dr. Shapiro's point was directed to the even larger pipeline issue in modern medical education, the lack of medical students choosing primary care as a specialty and going into practice. She continued:

The cost of a medical education today literally forces medical students, even the most altruistic and idealistic, to choose medical specialties that will allow them to pay back their student loans. And this generation is more into show and face. Glamour. I believe this also influences the kind of medicine they choose to practice. Endocrinology and primary care are *not sexy*. (speaker's emphasis).

Not sexy. When I told Dr. Shapiro that she wasn't the first person to mention that over the course of my research, she wasn't surprised:

It's really all about money, power, and sex. It's always been this way. But through all kinds of media people get this message at younger and younger ages. Medicine is no different. Students know it, they want it, [and] they get it.

In terms of professional prestige and financial reward, endocrinology and primary care, and for that matter, Type 2 diabetes, are not seen as low-hanging golden apples within the desired reach of U.S. medical school graduates and practitioners. The growing Type 2 diabetes and cardiometabolic population, from the perspective of professional labor, requires large numbers of trained physicians willing to address the demand side of this illness phenomenon. It is estimated that there are between 7,000 to 10,000 available endocrinologist positions in the United States.[44] As of 2019, the American Association of Clinical Endocrinologists (AACE) claims a membership of around 6,500 in the United States and ninety-nine other countries.[45] In short, the AACE's entire global membership is less than the estimated number of available endocrinologist positions in the United States alone.

At the Diabetes Teaching Center at the University of California, San Francisco, the CDEs are stretched thin, wearing many hats—as nurses, registered dieticians, clinicians, and pharmacists—in addition to their administrative and diabetes class and workshop planning duties. These professional duties and obligations spread them throughout the UC San Francisco medical complex. In effect, there are not enough CDEs available to meet growing patient demand for diabetes services, education, and community outreach. One CDE estimated that there are approximately 1.7 CDEs at UCSF to administer to the needs of the entire diabetes population served by the hospital.

Darlene Pedraza complained of gatekeeping within these understaffed hospitals (she was not referring to UCSF) where she unsuccessfully lobbied to start a diabetes education class. She believes that diabetes centers jealously guard their potential diabetes patients/students, particularly those with private health insurance. Public health CDEs such as her are left to scramble, organizing classes and workshops among the elderly, disenfranchised, and uninsured.

One day after class, a woman walked up to her, full of worry. "Darlene, my doctor referred me to a diabetes education class at _____ Hospital and I just found out that my health insurance was charged nine hundred dollars! I thought the class was free. What can I do?" Darlene recommended she take up the issue with her physician, insurance company, and the hospital. "This happens all too often," Darlene told me later, "Many physicians have no idea whether they are referring their patients to free public diabetes classes or fee-based ones."

The shortage of endocrinologists and CDEs points to another phenomenon in the Type 2 diabetic contemporary: a growing gendered division of labor in the delivery of services, education, and treatment. While endocrinologists are predominately male and as physicians can be imagined as a masculine form of embodied expertise, CDEs, on the other hand, coming mostly from the ranks of nurses, dieticians, and nutritionists, are overwhelmingly female.[46] I find this instructive in terms of analyzing the gendered role of both expertise and technology.

EXPERT BARRIERS TO EXPERTISE

Over the past two decades, there has been a renewed focus on patient-centered care. A 2001 Institute of Medicine (IOM) report identified patient-centered care as one of six interrelated factors constituting high-quality health care.[47] Patient-centeredness encourages eliciting patients' ideas, viewing patients and physicians as partners, and taking patients' emotional and social environments into account.[48] Patient-centeredness has been linked with increased patient satisfaction, improved patient outcomes, and more professionally fulfilled providers. This move toward patient-centered care has been challenged by the rapidly increasing cultural and social diversity of patients served coupled with the comparative lack of diversity among medical professionals. While not new, the corresponding need to teach cultural competence (CC) in health communication has become increasingly essential, but substantial pedagogical and practical challenges remain.[49] Only since the turn of the century has the idea of CC in medical education been a primary health communication goal.[50] Research examining student, resident, and attending physician attitudes about CC has raised questions about how to best implement CC training into the medical school curricula.[51] Other survey and data collection strategies have centered on subjective patient perceptions of their hospital care.[52]

Although CC curricula have been shown to increase student awareness, little is known about how this academic training is later implemented within the constraints and opportunities presented during clinical rounds.[53] Significantly, less is known about the social contexts and timings that frame possibilities for robust culturally competent teaching and learning between physicians, medical students, and patients. Earlier ethnographic research confounded this lack of understanding by situating CC pedagogy spatially within classroom and hospital conference rooms, seeing the bedside primarily as a knowledge dissemination endpoint.[54] Bedside teaching was viewed as a problematic ritual performance that affects both language and behavior.[55]

More recent ethnographic work examining teaching during clinical rounds has focused on communication between attendings and residents,[56] and bedside teaching as a contingent practice in which the implicit or "hidden" curriculum readily aligns itself with explicit curricular structures and models.[57] Ethnographic approaches provide context in charting both clinical and social change occurring over time.[58] As a pedagogical tool, one ethnographic approach, direct observation, has been recommended to medical faculty as a way of teaching students how "to watch closely from a distance."[59]

Although a plethora of cultural competency models and ethno-

graphic studies exist in the medical education and medical care arenas, little research has examined these models as *effective on-the-ground
practices generating improved patient-centered outcomes.*[60] The stakes in
question revolve around linking professional development in medical
schools and teaching hospitals with robust patient outcomes.[61] Medical practice, knowledge, and education could no longer be seen as "cul-
tureless" or "beyond culture."[62] Toward this goal of linking effective
professional development with improved patient outcomes, social and
behavioral science approaches to medical education emphasize that
cultural competence must be considered as a subset of any robust assessment of clinical competence.[63] Professionalism, an oft-conceived
innate character trait, requires a progressive redefinition: as a product
of dynamic development processes influenced by changing external
organizational structures and environmental contexts in both medical
practice and education.[64]

The CDC now recognizes the importance of understanding the
communities within which obesity, Type 2 diabetes, and other cardiometabolic disorders arise. Previously, the CDC's Community/Clinical
Partnership Model framed community and clinic as separate sectors.[65]
The Ecological Model, an outgrowth of the Healthy People 2010
program, initially placed undue emphasis on individuals instead of
communities, despite the fact that individuals are inseparable from
communities.[66] In other words, the physician/patient dyad served
as the focal point of programmatic attention, a relationship between
the clinic and the individual narrowed optically by a blurred exclusion of wider community contexts. Over a decade later, the Diabetes Prevention Program continues to face the challenge of translating
clinical research into viable community outreach programs.[67] Health
care and outreach professionals receive little to no training in effective
intercultural communication, thus making it more difficult to come
up with a coherent public outreach model that integrates the community and the clinic, particularly among diverse populations occupying
a singular racial category.[68] Therefore, efforts at recruitment must first
successfully train medical professionals as learners before any robust
culturally competent outreach to individuals, within clinics, and toward communities.

Merlene Bailey and I met for one of our early-morning breakfast
meetings at a local Rochester restaurant. Unkle Moe's, a veritable institution in the African American community, is located across the

street from the only remaining supermarket in Southwest Rochester's predominantly African American neighborhood.[69] Merlene sees important challenges in reaching out to historically segregated urban communities of color, particularly in the growing food deserts with limited access to fresh fruits and vegetables. Yet despite her position with the American Diabetes Association, membership in the Mt. Zion health cabinet, and years of experience in both diabetes clinical research and community education efforts, Merlene is not a CDE.

CDEs add to the calculus of how expertise is allocated and often rationed in communities throughout the Type 2 diabetic landscape. Despite a chronic shortage of CDEs, professional gatekeeping reveals the lucrative allure of the diabetes population as a growing market of consumers and patients. At the beginning of this century, in the face of an expanding Type 2 diabetes epidemic and market, the American Association of Diabetes Educators (AADE) restricted member eligibility to health professionals and away from community health workers.[70] Since then, Merlene says, she has received some resistance:

> No, I'm not a CDE, but I continue the work. I ask the Certified Diabetes Educators who have a problem with this several questions: One, why don't I see you in the communities that I work with? Two, do you understand, know how to communicate with, and make comfortable that *one African American* who shows up to your diabetes education class? Do you understand *where they are coming from?*

EXPERTISE THAT LISTENS AND LEARNS

A physician from West Africa who did her residency in the United States during the height of the 1980s crack cocaine epidemic lent credence to Merlene Bailey's assertions:

> I saw conditions in Baltimore that reminded me of conditions in Liberia. Clinicians often misread and misrecognized African American patients suspiciously. I was asked to translate and make legible the cultural dissonance clinicians had about African Americans. I'm not from Baltimore, or the U.S., but here I am being asked [to understand], and as it turned out, actually understood, African American patients better than nonblack clinicians. I realized that if they only *listened* to people, cultural competence

could be achieved. But they didn't. Although I had been bitten by the research bug, I found myself gravitating necessarily to patient advocacy and activism. (speaker's emphasis)

Merlene Bailey's emphatic questions interrogate and Dr. Johnson's statements disrupt the spatial *where* and the methodological *how* of public health outreach as much as the biomedical *what,* the individual *who,* or the social *why* of trust. Their insights concerning the relationships between clinic, community, and the role of missing experts raise the crucial issue of developing fluent biocommunication that can shift between and among different sociocultural registers without judgment.[71] Of critical importance, Merlene's fluency moves between different linguistic registers of a diverse black population, from African American Vernacular English to West Indian Creole English, and Standard English. For example, she shifted seamlessly between registers in warning audiences about the unreliability and potential danger of using "bush," or herbs, in attempting self-treatment for diabetic symptoms, as well as distinguishing *yam* from *sweet potato.*[72]

Other local knowledges around herbal remedies that Merlene Bailey recognizes also coincided with Dr. Asela's experiences in Sri Lanka. His eyes lit up when I mentioned *karwila* (*Momordica* spp., which includes bitter melon and balsam pear: *karavellaka* in Sanskrit, *karela* in Hindi, *caraille* in the Eastern Caribbean, *cerasee* in Jamaica), a bitter herb prescribed in South Asian Ayurvedic medicine for hyperglycemia, or elevated blood sugar levels. In sync, *cerasee* was one of the "bush" medicines Merlene warned her Afro-diasporic audience against.[73] I had previously spent a year in India and Sri Lanka visiting Ayurvedic medical colleges and pharmacies. Dr. Asela once recounted the many mornings his mother forced him to drink an infusion of bitter *karwila.* He then quickly seized hold of himself, his wistful recollection ending abruptly: "We must remember that traditional medicines are useful only in self-limiting illnesses; meaning, conditions which would have eventually resolved themselves over the course of time."

However, it was apparent that Dr. Asela was quite proud of the materia medica, knowledge production, and therapeutic practices developed in Ayurveda over two millennia in Sri Lanka. Sri Lankan Ayurveda, too, had its religious foundation in Buddhist monasteries and temples, medical colleges, and hospitals.[74] Dr. Asela came from Sri Lanka to upstate New York to practice biomedicine and in the process became aware of the health, educational, and economic disparities of urban America. It is in this and other zones of health disparity that Merlene Bailey, Dr. Johnson, Dr. Asela, and others seek to cultivate relationships through outreach toward African American and other at-risk communities.

In contrast, Merlene Bailey's facility in linguistic shifting fully conveyed both cultural content and social knowledge, and not merely changes in accent, dialect, or diction—something Dr. Johnson quickly attuned to but Dr. Asela still struggled to access through partnering within African American religious spaces. According to Merlene, not only were CDEs missing in action, but when found, they were unable to hold a community-wide conversation and make a community-wide difference because they lacked effective cross-cultural communication aptitudes for reaching diverse African American communities. She extended her critique of the lack of cultural competence to the local university hospital and medical center: "They like to invite the community up to say, 'This is who we are and this is what we have,' but they know little about *us*."

Merlene's comment points to the need for health professionals and community health workers attuned to the demographic particularities of diverse communities who often occupy a singular racial category. Professional, academic, and class structures may make claims to and erect gates around the siloed term *expert*. Nonetheless, *expertise* can be learned and copied, informed by the relatively unfettered community access and cultural competence of the community health worker. Dr. Johnson demonstrated that physicians could also acquire CC expertise, not as speaking experts in monologue but as listening learners in dialogue. The cultural diversity of the African American racial category requires broadening the notion of expertise from undifferentiated monocultural competence to a multiculturally fluent professional competence. Although churches may appear a logical repository of black diversity, several important demographic factors limit their usefulness as venues for outreach to the larger at-risk community.

THE LIMITS OF ENGENDERING TRUST THROUGH THE BLACK CHURCH

Studies focusing on the relationship between religion and African American health participation reveal skewed gender and age ratios.[75]

In these studies, participants who are predominantly female and over forty years of age tend to reflect church, not community, demographics. Similarly, at the workshop, there were more African Americans at Mt. Zion (fifty-three) than at the eight previous diabetes workshops and classes that I attended at the Clinical Research Center combined (two). Further, most attendees at the Mt. Zion workshop appeared to be forty years of age and older, with women comprising the overwhelming majority (thirty-nine versus fifteen) of those present.

Moreover, the rise of the "prosperity" gospel over the last three decades has elicited critical debate in many black churches, mirroring concerns in the wider society about the divine ordainedness of material and gustatory good fortune.[76] Local money and sex scandals in Rochester involving African American clergy did nothing to diminish speculation about where money came from, where money went, and the forms of suburban salvation it furnished. The relative lack of church attendance also reveals that many church-absent younger males and females tend to place trust in seeking future salvation elsewhere.

Three demographic particularities condition the possibility of instrumentalizing religion to achieve robust public health outreach and research recruitment goals within church spaces. First, larger socioeconomic, cultural, and structural issues stratify the "black church" by age and gender in ways that exclude younger and overwhelmingly male members of the community peripheral to church participation.[77] Second, of noticeable concern, youth and young adults of color have increasingly achieved diabetes control and other forms of primary medical care in penal institutions.[78] Third, and most notably, while a minor presence in both church participation and church-based public health outreach, African American males harbor the least amount of trust in biomedical research of any single demographic group.[79] That said, during my course of research I found no program that successfully brought youth and young adults into these Type 2 diabetes outreach efforts.

The existential facts of black life and death often demand more immediate, more pragmatic concerns that can make notions of Type 2 seem theoretical in the abstract. Rochester, New York, is a predominantly African American urban area, where, in extremis, both "race" and urbanity combine to ensure that an African American male will die, on average, twenty-one years earlier than an Asian American female living on the west coast of the United States.[80] As of 2007, Southwest

Rochester and the adjacent Maple Neighborhood bordering Eastman Kodak's main offices had an African American male homicide rate seventy times the national average.[81] In 2012, Rochester, the fifth poorest urban area in the United States, had the lowest African American male high-school graduation rate in the nation.[82] It was scarcely imaginable during the days of Jim Crow that urban areas such as Rochester would, in the future, prove more deleterious to African American health than the contemporary rural Southern United States.[83]

TRUSTING IN SWEET SALVATION

Given the historical hubris of sacrificial exchange, I suggest that for African Americans, trusting in potential avenues to a salvageable future requires a certain alacrity and sense of discrimination. However, discrimination also has several definitional connotations: discriminating, both "racially" and in terms of judgment, a search to separate fact from fiction, sometimes with the help of a racially concordant interlocutor. For example, African American diabetes educators, patients, ministers, and physicians repeatedly expressed to me the value of, to paraphrase, "more black expertise in this area," and that "We need more people like you doing this work." What I found most surprising was the noticeable degree to which these comments and embedded sentiments intersected socioeconomic, education, age, gender, and geographic lines. Trust, I discovered, was thin on the ground. Innovative diabetes science, advanced technological precision, and pharmaceutical efficacy, as social forms of knowledge and social modes of exchange, were not seen as neutral or bias-free. In struggling to grasp "the context of the medical," the inclination to trust may prove difficult for those anticipating interactional bias when engaging often-obscure knowledge forms and institutional practices.[84]

Anthropological debates originating in the late nineteenth and early twentieth centuries also engaged the nexus between race, trust, and salvation. However, this "salvage anthropology" situated its theoretical narrative squarely within evolutionary ideologies and triumphant orientations of scientific and theological salvation, their respective roles in the Christian mission of the West, and the inevitable disappearance of "native" societies around the world.[85] In the scholarly absence of any sustained vertical engagement with the question of power and its horizontal social effects, cultivating trust among native populations was a prime objective of earlier colonial, missionary, and anthropological projects.[86] Medicine, often embedded within these respective and often overlapping projects, composed part of the investigatory and translational toolkit employed in the field.[87] Indeed, early to mid-twentieth-century scholarship on trust building through forms of exchange among "natives" has proven foundational to the social scientific canon.[88] In the early twenty-first century, anthropological scholarship, like biomedicine and public health, focuses on community and field settings within larger neoliberal structures of corporate and institutional ethics.[89]

Given both the history of Tuskegee and Merlene Bailey's illustrative case of the community health worker as *both* expert and cultural intermediary, I found myself both sympathetic to and troubled by these distrustful sentiments. On the one hand, I was troubled that the racial concordance used to facilitate the trust necessary for building research and community partnerships has gone indefensibly wrong in the past and could again in the future. On the other hand, I understood that trust is hard won, often tinged with hope, and an asymmetrical, negotiated effort to separate empirical facts from social facts. To trust is to admit vulnerability in seeking knowledge and care. It is a gesture of considerable faith and courage, an unsure study in reciprocation, and an attempt to stand firmly on the uneven terrain of social justice and unequal health outcomes. Trust is not merely a cognitive but also a material artifact of history, reciprocity, and affect, in which epistemic differences are inevitably produced and contingently bridged.[90]

THE CHURCH AS A HIERARCHICAL SOCIAL NETWORK

W. E. B. Du Bois wrote in 1903 that the Negro church was an "organization . . . a remnant of African tribal life."[91] He argued that it was the singular mode of expressing slaves' "organized efforts," and "*any movement* among freedmen should centre about their religious life."[92] Social reform and racial uplift intersected with evolutionary discourses about Christianity and the civilizational fitness of African Americans for assuming their rights to full citizenship. Yet as a reflection of society, churches vary in terms of wealth and social status, as well as the cultural, educational, and professional pedigree of their congregants. Few churches, particularly African American congregations, can boast among their members a former mayor, a television news anchor, and high-level managers like Merlene Bailey of the American Diabetes Association and Robert Mann from the Alzheimer's Association.

Mt. Zion highlights the black church not as a monolith, but as a hierarchical social network demonstrating important links between voice and venue in establishing trust, something clinical research and public health actors now recognize yet struggle to articulate cogently in these spaces. As a form of exchange, trust is relational but not relative. These relationships serve to reproduce power, difference, and the social order. While outreach efforts centering on diabetes and its associated risk factors face the challenge of successfully targeting the younger generation, such projects through churches often occur within food deserts such as Southwest Rochester, illustrating the structural challenges involved in eliminating intergenerational health disparities. Amid these realities, the contexts of people's lives make the struggle more difficult. The larger collective challenge is how to effect positive metabolic change en masse, all the more so within unsafe and aesthetically depressed areas marked by resource deprivation, spatial segregation, mass incarceration, and myriad forms of socioeconomic disparity. Conversely, gentrification necessitates ongoing ethnographic attention to the ways shifting neighborhood demographics rationalize new biomedical entreaties to trust among rapidly reconfiguring communities and religious formations. From the standpoint of social and medical justice, that would offer new analytical avenues for examining whether biomedical and public health projects can build ethical reciprocity sustainably along and beyond the categorical intersections of race, class, gender, and generation.

As the twenty-first century ensued, the thorny matter of trust would continue to spark debate about the role of African-descent populations in biomedical research. The decoding of the human genome at the turn of the century molecularized race, "Africa," and gender, while bringing into sharper focus the ways in which research inclusion and participation highlighted historical forms of unequal social exchange and wealth production. These developments, as we shall explore next, promised to help researchers better understand the biological mechanisms driving Type 2 diabetes as well as the wider cardiometabolic constellation of illnesses. But more importantly, the genomic era reawakened intersecting discourses about race, gender, and bioethics, this time not only about those subjects and data points boxed within a racial category, but also among researchers of color imbricated within the research enterprise. Under the neoliberal banner of *diversity,* nature, science, and society offered new rationales for making claims that sub-Saharan DNA held the skeleton key to unlocking the metabolic doors to life itself. Introductory entreaties to recruit the *Other,* "without worrying their patience," would have to take on new form in offering novel sermons of salvation from pathological sweetness.

The Ascension of the Black Matriarch

THE SEARCH FOR METABOLIC AFRICA

> Pharma is a reflection of us, whites. But our company, like the [rest of the] U.S., is realizing that we can't just focus on the majority population and those with power and money. We now have a scientific basis for overseas trials—this is where genetics come in. We have to argue that different diseases originate in different ways in different people. This is a new way to look at diversity.
>
> —Pharmaceutical company executive, 2010

> No idea is more provocative in controversies about technology and society than the notion that technical things have political qualities.
>
> —Langdon Winner, *The Whale and the Reactor*

In July 2000, *Time* published a cover story celebrating the work of Craig Venter and Francis Collins for successfully sequencing the human genome.[1] Heralded as a scientific breakthrough comparable to Watson and Crick's discovery of DNA, the mapping of the human genome portended a future both of greater therapeutic hope for some and for others, one of biological dread. It seemed as if the secrets of life had finally yielded to scientific investigation and that the tinkering was about to begin. However, by 2009, a much more subdued optimism prevailed. "The publication of the highest-quality and best-annotated personal genome yet tells us much about sequencing technology, something about genetic ancestry, but still little of medical relevance."[2] In 2010, Venter himself stated, "We have learned nothing from the human genome." He saw no short- or medium-term applicability of genomic research to improving medical outcomes.[3]

Up to this point, the book has focused in broad historical and social scientific terms on African-descent recruitment and participation in biomedical research and public health imaginaries of race. The basis of this focus, the global production of sweetness through African bodies racialized by capital, extends to the search for genetic triggers of Type 2 diabetes in the ancestral past of precapital, preslavery, sub-Saharan diversity and presweetened African bodies. More boldly, if DuBois's "color-line" represented the overriding social problem of the twentieth century, I argue in the following that "diversity" represents the overriding social problem of the twenty-first. And like the color-line, diversity as a social problem radiates inward toward and outward from political, scientific, and historical contact points in coproducing both science and society.

This chapter continues to explore recruitment through the lens of race. But I pivot to how race came to represent "diversity" since the genomic research moment at the turn of the century, when the metabolic history of the world began retracing its narrative steps back to sub-Saharan Africa and the role African-descent populations could play in providing an alphabet for telling the story. Tracing metabolic ancestry back to sub-Saharan Africa takes our conversation, and this chapter's directionality, from race to gender, to shed light on how black women figure prominently in the new genomic moment, as researchers gaze into the maternally inherited fraction of DNA governing metabolism and environmental adaptation to, for our purposes, sweetness.

As this chapter proceeds, finding mitochondrial Africa in African American female bodies, as a novel exercise in inclusion, recruitment, and participation, raises perennial bioethical questions of consent and obligations to exchange. Genomic research provokes such an inquiry into the possibility of justice in the absence of reciprocation. From a social scientific perspective, I situate this inquiry into the possibility of justice within larger discourses of black matriarchy, matrifocality, and racial admixture.

I show that labor and capital produce diabetic bodies, rather than assume that race and gender, as kinship, reproduces diabetic risk. I aim to demonstrate the impartial universality of Type 2 diabetes risk in disproving notions of the Other's thrifty genes and the North Atlantic's presumed metabolic invincibility. We shall see that genomic *Af-*

rica as genomic diversity is alive and well in the New World, and why *she*, wearing an empty matriarchal crown bereft of power, has influenced the parameters of cardiometabolic research globally and utterly.

GENEALOGIES OF SCALE

The cost of sequencing a genome fell precipitously after I began my research project in 2008.[4] From 2008 to 2010, the cost to sequence an entire human genome dropped from US$100,000 to $4,400. In 2011, The National Human Genome Research Institute (NHGRI) released data collected by tracking the costs of genomic analysis during the period 2001–2011.[5] Further, these "second-generation" sequencing technologies perform greater coverage of a sequenced genome by "resequencing" the genome up to thirty or even forty times. This coverage sequencing (or "redundancy") permits a reliably high-quality reading of a genome.[6]

A human genome consists of the twenty-three chromosomal pairs of DNA representing around twenty thousand genes. Whole genomic sequencing analyzes the entire genome, reading each of the twenty thousand individual genes, scripted in the form of letters, known as *alleles*. The number of alleles is estimated at around three billion. This whole-genome analysis searches for genetic mutations or variants that may signal disease risk. However, the twenty thousand genes packaged within the twenty-three DNA chromosomal pairs comprise 99 percent of the genome. The remaining 1 percent of the genome contains a nongenetic material called an *exome*, which codes proteins within the genome. Some researchers see exomic research as the future of genetic investigations into disease causation, offering both greater cost-effectiveness and more useful data than whole-genome sequencing.[7]

The second-generation technologies precipitating the decline in genomic sequencing costs made exomic sequencing possible. The cost decline of genomic sequencing outpaced Moore's Law, which posits decreasing costs over time as technological advances result in a doubling of computing power every two years. "This facilitated the movement from genetics to genomics," said Dr. Mikel, a genetic/genomic researcher, when we spoke in 2010. "We can now increase the number of genomes we put through analysis, producing millions of sequences in a single run." Today with fourth-generation technologies, the economics of sequencing the human genome has carved new research space for investigating both human and disease origins. In the attempt to keep up with these rapidly emerging areas of research, the new suffix "-omics" has come to describe the ever-expanding range of genomic research attention. This includes research in epigenomics, which involves looking at recent environmental influences upon the genome; microbiomics, the genomics of gut bacteria; and metabolomics, the genomics of metabolism and energy regulation. Lastly, newer work in mitogenomics examines the function of maternally inherited mitochondrial DNA in tracing ancestry and ancient migration across the world.[8]

DIVERSITY AS RACE

In the face of these rapid technological developments, the National Institutes of Health (NIH) formed Genome-Wide Association Studies (GWAS) in 2008. GWAS was designed as both a database and a repository for the large amounts of genomic data emerging from sequencing technologies. A data-sharing hub, GWAS aimed to foster greater coordination of research activities and outcomes. The repository, known as dbGaP (Database of Genotype and Phenotype), contains data on unexpressed (genotypical) and expressed (phenotypical) traits found in different populations. However, according to GWAS, roughly 86 percent of genetic samples collected originate from those of European background.[9]

Genomic research over the last decade has mapped in greater detail the wide genetic diversity of sub-Saharan African populations. Recently, the genomic research on this Type 2 genetic complexity, known as the metabolic syndrome (MetS), has focused on examining mitochondrial (mt)DNA and its energy and metabolic system. Derived through maternal lines, mtDNA regulates energy production by utilizing oxygen to convert food to energy. This energy regulatory mechanism represents human adaptation to a diverse set of environmental, and this chapter argues, historical challenges.[10]

Given the multitude of factors contributing to the development of Type 2 diabetes, such as obesity, physical inactivity, and excess caloric intake, other approaches to the genetic study of the illness are being recommended. Diabetics usually die from heart disease, kidney disease, or stroke, with associated conditions such as hypercholesterolemia, hypertension, retinopathy, neuropathy, and other circulatory disorders. Therefore, scientific arguments posit that researching the genetic causes of MetS in its entirety would prove more productive than a singular focus on the genetics of Type 2 diabetes. The National Heart, Lung, and Blood Institute (NHLBI) Family Heart Study found genetic correlations to MetS biomarkers such as insulin resistance, waist circumference, hypertension, body mass index (BMI), HDL cholesterol, and triglycerides.[11] However, the authors stopped short of attributing disease causation solely to genetic factors, concluding, "These results suggest that pleiotropic effects of genes or shared family environment contribute to the familial clustering of MetS-related traits."[12] In other words, the researchers' ambiguous conclusion seemed unwilling to go beyond, much less settle, older discourses of nature versus nurture and biology versus culture, as it spawned newer conversations about genetics (DNA) versus epigenetics (mRNA) and genomics (mtDNA) versus epigenomics (mtRNA).

At the end of the first decade of the twenty-first century, the exploration for genetic sites of Type 2 diabetes causation had focused on small-scale studies that uncovered only two loci, which when mutated, produced only a monogenetic (single gene) form of the illness, not the complex form commonly seen clinically. Those meta-analytical study outcomes increased the number of potential loci discovered to forty-four. Researchers posited that investigating the genetic causes of MetS in its entirety would prove more productive than a simple focus on the genetics of Type 2 diabetes. Although that seemed promising, it represented only around 10 percent of all the potential clusters of high-risk families in Europe with Type 2 diabetes.[13]

Toward the end of the second decade of the century, advances in genomic sequencing technology permitted larger scale studies of Type 2 diabetes and the creation of polygenetic risk scores (PRS) that estimate diabetes risk based on risk profiles of dozens of genetic loci.[14] In spite of these developments, the reference libraries of genetic samples used in research still overwhelmingly originate from Euro-American populations. The Finnish, Danish, and Tethys examples illustrated how genetic homogeneity drove recruitment efforts to diversify their respective research sample bases. The relative absence of African genetic samples in the genomic archive strangely resembles earlier absences of African ancestries from the historical archive. The untold stories represent volumes of unrecorded history and ancestry: A 2019 study of 910 individuals of admixed and unmixed African descent from the Americas and continental Africa uncovered millions of genetic bases unaccounted for in the genomic reference library.[15] An earlier 2015 study, the 1000 Genomes Project, sampled 26 global populations, of which 5 originated in African populations. Those 5 African populations contained more genomic variation than the other 21 combined.[16]

Therefore, the approximately 86 percent of GWAS samples originating in European populations leave a wider genetic research world of Type 2 diabetes risk to explore. As of 2017, roughly 2 percent of the GWAS library contained African American/Afro-Caribbean samples, and an additional 0.57 percent originated from continental African groups. These represent a four- and twofold increase, respectively, since 2009, yet by number, both pale in comparison to the increase in Asian samples during that time.[17] The directionality of the genomic research gaze now eyes the wide genetic diversity of African-descent populations, along with South Asian and Native American populations in the effort to make new genomic associations with Type 2 diabetes. The inclusion of African-descent populations and others could help identify new areas of susceptibility, grow sample size, and improve predictive power. The diversity science moment has arrived.

The first part of this chapter explores health disparities in research recruitment organized around biological understandings of racially classified and stratified human populations. Otherwise known as *diversity,* these fragmented and stratified populations reveal the political history underpinning the biopharmaceutical assemblage itself. The second part of this chapter explores how race, gender, and ancestry confound genomic understandings of difference and disease, as well as the bioethical implications of diversity outreach for and translation of such research.

I borrow the term *diversity science* from one of my interlocutors to describe the knowledge production emerging from the recruitment of racial difference in genomic research and the unique yet problematic role African-descent populations play in these efforts. In this chapter, I present two interrelated examples: I begin with an ethnographic narrative outlining the imagined strategic role of diversity in pharmaceutical research. The second example describes how researchers in my project viewed U.S. African Americans both as a sub-Saharan African and an admixed population. In terms of racial recruitment, a new genomic scramble for Africa, not confined by geography but defined as biology, highlighted perennial bioethical questions of consent, participation, and justice. It did so in ways that push our discussion necessarily from race, or rather *through* race, to an examination of diversity rooted in specific sociocultural histories of gendered exchange and obligations to give, without necessarily producing equal obligations to reciprocate.

DIVERSITY SCIENCE

The mapping of the human genome sparked speculation about the possibility that the pharmaceutical development of drug targets, or new molecules designed to target specific genetic/genomic sites, might one day become realized. Indeed, nearly ten years before the Supreme Court decision in 2013 banning ownership of the human genome, the pharmaceutical industry initiated the patenting of genomic fragments in an accretive, piecemeal fashion that threatened to result in eventual ownership of a human genome under full patent and intellectual property-right protection. In 2009, Roche Pharmaceuticals acquired Genentech for an estimated US$47 billion. Roche saw coupling its pharmaceutical heft with Genentech's focus on genetic, genomic, and postgenomic research as a logical acquisition strategy. Costs associated with Type 2 diabetes continue to constitute the majority of the health care dollars spent by an illness population that comprises a dependable base of repeat consumers from increasingly diverse populations. Race, ethnicity, national character, and market strategies all play a role in what one of my interlocutors surmised as "big pharma reimagining its client base."[18]

In June 2011, I sat in a large conference hall filled with researchers, graduate students, and community health workers of color facing a panel of pharmaceutical company executives and representatives. We gathered in Houston to learn more about diversity issues both within pharmaceutical companies and in clinical research trials. The executives came to argue that diversity on both the inside and outside of pharmaceutical production lay at the core of reducing health disparities. The panel chair made it clear: "This panel is not the panel to address questions of price, profit, and promotion. We ask that we limit our discussion to the topic of health disparities and the potential role of pharma in helping address them." Nerves were definitely on edge in both sides of the hall.

The session began with an African research executive for a large firm stating, "Big pharma is criticized a lot about what we do, with some people calling it 'the dark side.' Instead, I sought to bring diversity to research, finding most studies comprising 90–95 percent Caucasians. I argued that something was wrong with this picture." Citing the need for what she called "diversity science," her company now has over two hundred research sites across the United States and has identified and formed partnerships with a multiethnic group of physician-researchers. The company began its "diversity science" project by hiring ten African American and Latino researchers each, relying on them to raise issues of need specific to their respective populations in helping fine-tune its research focus. As a result, the company then sought to hire two hundred each of African American, Latino, Chinese, and white researchers. Although the company reached their hiring goals for the other groups, they were only able to recruit sixty-seven African Americans. "We need more African American researchers to reach out to the African American population. We are aware of the experiences of African Americans in medical history. But I am here to tell you that pharma is learning to listen." I was not sure if what I had heard up to that point was tinged with humility, contrition, or even a hint of confession.

The second speaker, a nervously awkward executive from another large pharmaceutical firm, maintained this tone: "Pharma is a reflection of us, whites. But our company, like the [rest of the] U.S., is realizing that we can't just focus on the majority population and those with power and money. We now have a scientific basis for overseas trials— this is where genetics come in. We have to argue that different diseases originate in different ways in different people. This is a new way to look at diversity." She then jumped from genotype to phenotype, claiming that drugs work differently in different racial groups. She said that her company was in the process of developing a race-based drug and soberly outlined the role diversity plays in shaping corporate pharmaceutical and biotechnology mindsets:

> The population of the Unites States is becoming more diverse each year, with groups of people coming from areas of the world where drug companies are working in. Drug-company research in those areas of the world will not contract, but expand. Companies are becoming increasingly aware of the need for this offshore research in dealing with a changing U.S. population of medical consumers.

There should be no doubt that translating "ideas to income" remains central to pharmaceutical company objectives. Following the demise of race-based pharmaceuticals in the last decade, global projects today envision "diversity" as "pharmacogenomic variance." This rhetorical shift reflects DNA procurement efforts aimed at producing genetic target drugs for an increasingly diverse and economically important North Atlantic population.

Technological advances have contributed significantly to reimagining the market harnessing diversity as a resource. However, some African-descent researchers I spoke with had mixed opinions about the value of participating in genomic research. For Dr. Ralston, an African American geneticist, research inclusion constitutes a vital component of producing both knowledge and justice through "participation" by minorities, both as research subjects and researchers. "If we don't care enough about what is happening in our own families and communities, then who will?"

Dr. Ralston is one of a cohort of geneticists and molecular epidemiologists of color trained at historically black colleges and universities. Aware of the history of the Tuskegee Syphilis Study, he believes that custodianship of African-descent DNA is a matter of social justice and ethical responsibility. However, he saw attempts to collect this DNA as driven more by economic and scientific motives than a desire to reduce health disparities. He said, "I know a lot of people working in genomics. Trust me, most of them don't give a damn about black people. But they can't ignore the amounts of money coming into genomic research." Ralston's belief in the importance of African-descent sampling exists in historical tension with dual suspicions about the interests of the market and the curiosity of science. After all, both market interest and scientific curiosity have figured greatly in constructing the historical edifice of race. However, recruiting diversity also requires the use of old categorical understandings of racial and ethnic difference, while problematizing their exact genomic definition and location.

AFRICANICITY AND ADMIXTURE

I had landed in Raleigh-Durham. Building on contacts made and interviews conducted during summer 2011, in spring 2012 I attended the Genetics of the Peoples of Africa and the Transatlantic African Diaspora Conference, held at the University of North Carolina, Chapel

Hill. An international meeting, the conference brought together biological anthropologists, geneticists, molecular biologists, and epidemiologists of color whose work addressed the genetics of health or health disparities in transnational and diasporic African-descent populations. The meeting raised three important and contentious issues: one epistemic, one definitional, and one methodological. The first issue centered on personal identification within a "racial" or "ethnic" group. The second revolved around the definition of an "African." The third centered on locating "Africa" in the "admixed" human genome. It became clear that locating Africa on the genomic map was no less challenging than defining an African in racial terms. Diversity science as a racial project must contend with race as a product of history.

The auditorium was abuzz during the morning question-and-answer session. An African American molecular biologist, Dr. Marcus Scribner, who had participated in the Houston meeting I attended the year before, sought to contest the definition of an "African" as a member of a sub-Saharan group on the continent. This molecular biologist, visibly perturbed by the ways race had been linked to specific genomic scripts in an earlier presentation, presented an epistemic challenge: "Ancestry tests for ancestors, not living people. It is an act of categorical misrecognition to attempt to explain genetic and genomic differences within human populations using the language of race." Against efforts to define "an African" as a member of a sub-Saharan group on the continent, Scribner argued, "An African is someone who either originates from or lives within the African continent. It makes no difference whether what we call 'European' Y-chromosomes are found in North Africa, the U.S., and [sic] South Africa; or 'Arab' Y-chromosomes in the Sudan."

The biologist's comments point to a problem—actually, two big problems: the first centers on personal identification with a "racial" or "ethnic" group; the second revolves around the definition of an "African." Both problems originate in the sociopolitical histories, geographies, and economies of power that shape such identities. Scribner traced the assumptions behind such claims to nineteenth-century biological anthropology and evolutionary theory, which equated an exaggerated Bantu phenotype as the prototypical "Negro." "This was about Europe and America writing an evolutionary narrative to themselves about themselves and those below them as a result of contact, colonization and slavery. Knowledge produced for domestic consumption and the exercise of power, but wholly inaccurate."

Moreover, the historical dynamics of power challenge genomic narratives about race. One researcher who traces genomic ancestry in Latin America said,

> The population of the Dominican Republic has a heavy African component. In a continuum of *Africanicity,* from lowest to highest you have: Mexico, Ecuador, Colombia, Puerto Rico, and the Dominican Republic. Yet national and cultural narratives in the Dominican Republic focus on their "European heritage." Haitians are seen as the Africans although there are Dominicans with as much or more African genetic ancestry than Haitians.

Since the 1960s, several anthropologists and Afrocentric scholars have used the terms *Africoid* and *Africanicity* to describe an essential sub-Saharan-African aesthetic.[19] Over time, these two terms have been adopted by scholars in biological anthropology, diaspora studies, psychology, cultural studies, and increasingly, in the field of genetics. For example, *Africanicity* was deployed originally in studies of African art and film but is now taken up by some genomic researchers to describe degrees of sub-Saharan ancestry in a genetic sample.[20] What is unclear is precisely how and when the aesthetic became seen as biological, with some researchers using *Africanicity* to define a common "African American *cultural* DNA" (emphasis added), but the epistemic and definitional interpretations of African ancestry as biocultural deterritorialize sub-Saharan Africa geographically while simultaneously inferring its genetic locatability.[21] In anthropology, the racial science of the late nineteenth and twentieth centuries, and Herskovits's counterargument of a somatic Africa embedded within black bodies that remember, found linguistic allies but perhaps not political affines through the language of what some call *bio-Africanity.*[22]

Therein lay another problem, a historical one with biological, and now genetic, interpretations: that of diversity itself. Coded bioscientific languages of diversity and admixture coexist problematically with older social scientific terms equally rooted in essentialist thought. In the social sciences, humanities, and cultural studies, scholars use words such as *hybridity, mixing, assimilation,* and *creolization.* In biological terms, *natural selection, genetic drift, founders' effect,* and others come to mind. Sometimes, the biological and social terms are used interchangeably. Politically, *integration* and *multiculturalism* symbolize the interactive diversity of neoliberal democracy in the contemporary public sphere. However, in population genetics and genomics, *admixture* describes this biological synthesis. The "act of categorical misrecognition" Dr. Scribner referred to repeated the conceptual mistakes of the past: the presumption that two or more "pure types" *mixed*, a presumption that repeats the conceptual errors made in earlier scholarship on creolization.

The central question, therefore, remains: How to source the wide genetic diversity of sub-Saharan Africanicity in admixed African-descent populations? As one molecular epidemiologist told me,

> It is extremely difficult to source [African] origins in an admixed population. And of course, there can be degrees of admixture even within the same population. The Southeastern United States has the least racially admixed and the Pacific Northwest the most racially admixed African American populations in the United States. Testing Afro-Caribbean and Afro-Brazilian populations can perhaps tell us more about African ancestry than U.S. African Americans—too much admixture.

Admixture is both a problem and an opportunity for science. As an opportunity, for example, with the PreDX™ Diabetes Risk Score, the inclusion of undifferentiated African-descent populations and others could help identify new "susceptibility loci," grow sample size, and improve power.[23] Africanicity is the motherlode, figuratively and literally. The challenge involves the inevitable racialization that such an ancestral gaze invites. Moving backwards in physiological time, one would think that genetic/genomic explanations of difference could serve to mediate confusion about race, ancestry, and disease. The problem for genomic science rests in quantifying degrees of admixture when the only signifiers, or tools, for articulating difference remain embedded in older languages and assumptions about race.[24] Linking the genetics of race to the epidemiology of race poses another degree of explanatory difficulty.

To illustrate, genomic-admixture mapping endeavors to uncover how genetic ancestry influences disease risk. However, it relies upon older classificatory language—e.g., "European," "Native American," "African," "Asian," etc.—in the search for the genetic defects/effects of these ancestries upon the health of admixed individuals and populations. In 1997, the NIH mandated that all research data submitted be classified according to race. However, those classifications depend on the self-reported racial identity of the individual. As one researcher told me, "Garbage in, garbage out—we get what our categories restrict and allow." However, admixture mappers say the technology offers the opportunity to create two maps: one according to the self-identification of individuals, and another based on the actual percentages of ethnic and geographic ancestry in the same individual.

According to Dr. Barrington, "The high percentage of European Y-chromosomes in the African American population makes mitochondrial DNA a better locus of study. It is a circular genome that is maternally derived. It performs no recombination, is traceable, and more copies of it are available for study." Dr. Barrington's comment favoring genomic studies focusing on African American maternal lines through mtDNA analysis coheres with the gendered social history in the United States concerning interracial relationships. Whether by historical accident or scientific coincidence, finding Africa in all its sub-Saharan diversity and hence potential resources, in a U.S. population, involves, in terms of statistical success, an investigation of mtDNA through African-descent maternal lineages.

GENDERED AND RACIAL DIRECTIONALITIES

Over the last two decades, genomic research has illustrated with greater detail the wide genetic diversity of sub-Saharan populations. Mitochondrial DNA (mtDNA) is derived only through maternal lines, and the genetic information it contains regulates energy production by utilizing oxygen to convert food to energy. This energy regulation mechanism represents human adaptation to a diverse set of environmental and historical challenges. African Americans have some of the highest rates of Type 2 diabetes in the United States. However, their mtDNA contains diverse sets of sub-Saharan DNA. The genetic complexity of Type 2 diabetes includes cofactors that usually accompany the disease, including hypertension; hypercholesterolemia; eye, kidney, and heart diseases; chronically high blood sugar levels; and Alzheimer's disease. As mentioned previously, diabetics rarely die from diabetes itself but rather from one or more of these cardiometabolic factors. Recently, the genomic research focus on this Type 2 genetic complexity, known as the metabolic syndrome (MetS), has centered on examining mtDNA and its energy and metabolic system.[25]

On one hand, both admixture and Africanicity present unique challenges. On the other, they highlight the possible role of U.S. African Americans in genomic research. First, the United States was the only slave society that experienced a natural increase in its African-descent population. Caribbean slave economies like Jamaica, for example, preferred working slaves to death and replacing them with new imports from Africa.[26] By 1830, U.S. slaves, on average, already had three maternal ancestral generations preceding them who were born in the United States. From an epigenetic standpoint, African Americans, representing a diverse population in terms of admixture, demonstrate a longer history of genetic interaction with European populations. In terms of Africanicity, this population also demonstrates a predictable pattern of mtDNA flow through West African maternal lines. Just as important, and also relevant beyond the United States, enslaved African populations also represent relatively recent histories of intensive intra-sub-Saharan interaction as well.[27]

The ethical histories of scientific research involving African-descent populations in the Atlantic Rim and beyond perennially reemerged in Raleigh during these presentations, discussions, and subsequent interviews. At the same time, the effects of past historical, social, and health inequalities also elicited new concerns about future social and health disparities, if African-descent populations were not enrolled in genomic research. African Americans have some of the highest rates of Type 2 diabetes in the United States; however, their mtDNA contains diverse sets of sub-Saharan DNA. Recently, the genomic research focus on MetS has been centered on examining mtDNA, and its energy and metabolic system. Further, as we shall see, decoding admixture is not an insurmountable problem; *Africa* could be sourced within admixed bodies—and already had been for over half a century.

Older anthropological and sociological preoccupations with diversity among bodies now shared research attention with genetic diversity within bodies. The mapping of the human genome mirrored, in microcosm, the earlier mapping of the geographic world, the scientific quandaries of encounter, and the attendant politics of explaining diversity within hierarchical constructs of racial difference. Our concern remains embedded in the argument that race, gender, and genetics cannot tell stories outside of history. Mitochondrial DNA not only provides a lens for examining how metabolic adaptation to environmental change occurs but also makes a bioethical claim to justice based on historical forms of racial and gendered injustice, and why telling untold stories make those bioethical breaches legible. In the twenty-first century, understanding the mechanisms responsible for the development of Type 2 diabetes involved older questions about informed consent, the research gaze on the black and female body, and myriad ways value has been found, historically, in black bodies.

THE ASCENSION OF THE BLACK MATRIARCH

In a letter to the journal *Nature* on August 8, 2013, a research team led by Andrew Adey, Joshua Burton, and Jacob Kitzman from the Department of Genome Sciences at the University of Washington in Seattle announced the successful mapping of the genome and epigenome of the HeLa cell line.[28] This development occurred less than seven months after a German research group directed by Lars Steinmetz published data in an open access journal detailing the first successful genomic sequencing of a HeLa cell line.[29] These accomplishments promised to change the way researchers understood environmental adaptation and energy regulation as metabolic processes of genetic mutation. This advance could possibly shed new light on the causative factors and mechanisms underlying the development of Type 2 diabetes and other cardiometabolic disorders.

However, the international research community, particularly the National Institutes of Health, harbored concern about what the new discovery might mean for future research. Although the German team removed the online data, the family of Henrietta Lacks, who was the original source of the HeLa line, was especially concerned about the ethical implications of these discoveries. It seemed the scientific community was once again producing wealth and knowledge from the HeLa cell line without acknowledging its fraught history of bodily appropriation. As chronicled by Hannah Landecker and Rebecca Skloot, the HeLa cell line was commodified without the knowledge of Lacks's family at a time when informed consent was not yet a legal norm.[30] This time, however, the Lacks family demanded economic justice.

In a statement released the day before the announcement, Francis

Collins, director of the NIH, sought to reconcile the newly mapped HeLa line with the Lacks's demands:

> Just like their matriarch, the Lacks family continues to have a significant impact on medical progress by providing access to an important scientific tool that researchers will use to study the cause and effect of many diseases with the goal of developing treatments.[31]

On closer reading, the statement "Just like their matriarch, the Lacks family continues to . . . provid[e] access" reveals a vexed engagement with HeLa's history. Although Henrietta Lacks's consent to the use of her cervical cancer cells beyond the diagnosis and treatment of her condition was not required, the phrase "providing access" implies that she did. Collins's statement frames the family as a biological resource and locates labor value squarely within researcher expertise, reproducing HeLa's history of racialized and gendered forms of labor, kinship denial, and commodification that are often disavowed. Together, these issues make the intersections between genomics, race, and gender a fundamentally bioethical relationship.

Engaging with scientific and media narratives about Henrietta Lacks and HeLa, this section charts the ways genomic research has facilitated the reemergence of a particularly thorny term: *matriarchy.* Within the bioethical nexus of genomics, race, and gender, the invocation of matriarchy in these narratives makes the private "public," a process Karla Holloway argues constitutes a control of race and gender.[32] Hence, such scientific and media narratives belie racialized gender constructs based on African descent rooted in socioeconomic history, which I term *bioethical matriarchy.* This socioeconomic history reveals the absent political and resource allocations erased by the matriarchal label. In this sense, investigating bioethical matriarchy departs from Max Weber's century-long call for an analysis of technology separate from an analysis of the "property relations" among economic actors.[33]

I wish here to widen the discussion of the social facts driving racialized participation in Type 2 diabetes research to make two arguments: (1) Although race and gender have occupied much scholarly and media attention, matriarchy, specifically black matriarchy, as both a racial and gender construct of otherness, has remained underanalyzed yet routinely deployed in the social sciences, politics, and humanities;

(2) Underlining patriarchal gift economies of exchange, bioethical matriarchy (or the bioethical matriarch) marks racialized and gendered forms of exchange arising from the absence of consent or of obligational precedents for reciprocation. Four fundamental questions drive this inquiry: (1) What do novel matriarchal genomic origin narratives tell us about embedded racialized and gendered forms of exchange and their historical intersections with socioeconomic status and inequality? (2) How are race, gender, and the social order reproduced or regenerated as a productive economic construct? (3) How then might Type 2 diabetes reflect the reproduction and regeneration of the social order as a productive economic construct? (4) Therefore, can restorative or reparative justice render the bioethical matriarch healthy and whole? In other words, can justice, however framed, recover the memories of mothers lost, heal communities fractured, and safeguard against future thefts of black bodies?

Arguably, these questions matter, as the bioethical matriarch is positioned as not whole. Henrietta Lacks's matriarchal status derives not from any real power Lacks may have had, but from HeLa's subsequent notoriety gained recursively as a fragmentary biospecimen, while recentering sub-Saharan Africa metabolically in an admixed African American woman. I suggest that deconstructing the matriarchal-status ascription addresses the intersections of genomics, racial labor, and gender beyond their component social, political, and biological parameters. The recruitment of the inherited mechanisms driving pathological sweetness answers whether the political and economic power (dis)enfranchising inherited rights to resources accrue to the matriarch as a result of this exchange. The 2013 mapping of the HeLa genome and epigenome rewrote the conditions of exchange regarding the ethical recruitment of and the required criteria for gaining informed consent from prospective research participants.

RECRUITING CONSENT

The publication of the genomic and epigenomic map of HeLa prompted an urgent meeting at the NIH in August 2013, followed by another at the NHGRI in September 2013.[34] Ethical research recruitment and conduct protocols, codified in 1992 as the Common Rule, proved antiquated amid the rapidly advancing realities of genomic science in the early twenty-first century. Although calls for revisiting and revising the Common Rule had been made over the course of the preceding decade, the public notoriety concerning Henrietta Lacks's story and its attendant reverberations through her family forced the NIH's hand in finally rescripting a bioethical document that reset the ground rules for research inclusion and informed consent.[35]

The Belmont Report, written in the wake of the Tuskegee Syphilis Study that had ended officially only six years earlier in 1973, made recommendations for the future ethical recruitment of research participants, their rights therein, and the appropriate conduct of researchers thereof. Seeking an ethical evolute that both reinforced and transcended appropriate researcher behavior post-Nuremberg, the Belmont panel focused more squarely on the rights of research participants, while mindful of Tuskegee's blatant violations of the post–World War II Nuremberg Protocols and subsequent Helsinki Declaration in 1964. The Belmont authors urged the wholesale incorporation of their consensus report into future policy, from which the Common Rule implemented, but not in its entirety.[36]

Belmont stood on the three pillars of post-Nuremburg ethics: (1) the voluntary right to consent, (2) favorable benefits outweighing risks, and (3) the right to withdraw from research participation without repercussion.[37] Of note, the justification of "benefits" applied definitionally to individuals and/or society, but not to communities.[38] In her retrospective assessment of the Belmont Report, former panel member Patricia King expressed disappointment that she and colleagues' Belmont Committee post-Tuskegee bioethics foci on autonomy/individualism and consent excluded a thorough contextual interrogation of social justice.[39]

The 1992 Common Rule emerged as a result of the findings of the Belmont Report of 1979.[40] The 1980s had witnessed an increased outsourcing of pharmaceutical research. Growing populations of bioliterate Westerners and cosmopolitans had reduced the numbers of tractable test subjects for the growing research demands of the U.S. pharmaceutical industry. Research ethics became an offshore concern, negotiable with foreign governments, forged into a workable document. Market ethics tended to overrule both state protection and research ethics, and human subject protection protocols masked the contextual asymmetries of power and socioeconomic inequality in which clinical trials researchers worked.[41]

Neither "race" nor "gender" found mention in the Belmont Report, despite Tuskegee's egregious antecedence and HeLa's proliferation in the quarter century since Henrietta Lacks's death. Race and gender, as social and biological attributions of kinship respectively, do battle on the field of social justice: Recruiting and researching inherited risk each make insufficient the notion of the autonomous, consenting individual and require a rethinking of the ways families, communities, and social groups exist differentially and unequally in the bioscientific imagination. Such a rethinking demands a wider justification of benefits and risks beyond abstract framings of the individual and society, a rethinking that psychology, sociology, and anthropology continue to grapple with as well.

Arguably, bioethical preoccupations with the individual form part of a longer genealogy rooted in humanistic ideals that developed during the Enlightenment. The paradigmatic changes resulting from lifting the ban concerning dissection after the French Revolution changed notions of disease causation, death, the body, and the state. What Michel Foucault termed *anatomo-clinical* medicine shifted the therapeutic locus of medical interaction from the social space of the family home toward the clinic, and its social focus shifted from the family/patient dyad to the doctor/patient one. The social gaze became the medical gaze; advantageously, government(s) found a new means of surveillance and management of subject bodies.[42]

Deborah Gordon initiated a fruitful three-decade-long conversation situating Western naturalism and individualism at the heart of biomedicine.[43] Gordon argues that biomedical practices reinforce individualism and social atomization, which rest at the foundations of the West's ethos. The individual self, as a subject, by this definition, has become a historically informed reductionism in medical practice through its determining gaze on the body and its physiology. The anatomical atlas does not stand for the body: the anatomo-clinical revolution complete, the individual body now stands for it. It represents an epistemology and praxis of applied alienation that has reconfigured the body and identity, contributing to notions of liberalism, rational choice, and individual contract.[44]

Bioethical history has demonstrated that a medical gaze fixated upon the anatomized individual as the alpha and omega of consent and agency may have contributed to the alienation of the body from the family, community, and its categorical ascription. HeLa raises the historical stakes by moving the ethical goalposts from the gross anatomy of the sub-Saharan African to that of the mitochondrial bioenergetics of sub-Saharan Africa itself. Therefore, in terms of consent, HeLa extends bioethics beyond the individual, to the family, the community, and the category, and in so doing, rendered the Belmont Report presciently artefactual, the 1992 Common Rule effectively outdated, and the 2013 Revision to the Common Rule ethically controversial.

The ethical controversy centered on whether the 2013 Revision's continuing emphasis on individual autonomy overshadowed ethical protections for communities. Robust and convincing research data generation, particularly in the age of big data and its filtering through ethnoracial and gendered categories, depends statistically on large population sizes. Deidentification of individuals' biodata, safeguarded as an ethical protection, obviates the fact that individuals belong to communities and that communities, as shown in this book, serve as microcosmic examples of populations, variously categorized.[45] Mirroring the earlier discussion of the CDC's Community/Clinical Partnership, Ecological Model, Healthy People 2010 Program, and the Diabetes Prevention Program (DPP), the aftermath of the 2013 Revision, some argue, inadequately situates ethics, informed consent, and justice between the individual, the clinic, and the community.[46] It is in these still-undefined and blurred bioethical spaces that Dr. Asela, Tethys, and diversity science seek to recruit African Americans, only to find that unaddressed questions of justice and trust persist within Othered communities stratified historically, nearly seven decades after Framingham's original, now seemingly naïve, urging.[47] Nuremberg, Tuskegee, Belmont, and both incarnations of the Common Rule moved with incremental awakening toward the realization that the entire research enterprise of scientific knowledge production depends in large part on the historical conditions of unequal exchange that reproduce society, race, and gender.

DECONSTRUCTING MATRIARCHY, REPRODUCING SOCIETY

The *Oxford English Dictionary* defines a matriarch as "a woman who is the head of a family or tribe," and "an older woman who is powerful within a family or organization." Further, it defines matriarchy as "a system of society or government ruled by a woman or women." Discursively figuring Henrietta Lacks as "matriarch" positions her as a notable figure in her family, but this positioning elides her actual power in both her personal, family life (which we may not have access to) and larger cultural, historical, and social contexts reproducing dominant notions of race and gender.

Discursive framings of matriarchy in social and political scientific literatures have long labeled African American and, by extension, Afro-Creole family structures as "matriarchal," "matrilineal," or "matri-focal."[48] Moreover, invocations of matriarchy have usually contained political motivations.[49] For example, the 1965 Moynihan Report attributed "matriarchal" family structures to "the culture of poverty" affecting a large percentage of the African American population. Low rates of marriage, skewed representations in popular culture, and statistics on out-of-wedlock births reinforced the notion of endemic African American cultural pathology and family disintegration. And this biosocial "fact" of African American matriarchy has seeped into genomic discourse.

According to Lisa Weasel, the story of Henrietta Lacks reignited evolutionary debates about human origins, while reinscribing a narrative "from which race and gender cannot be extricated."[50] Race, a theoretical and methodological preoccupation of nineteenth- and early-twentieth-century biological anthropology that sought to find its essence, later gave way to cultural and postmodern arguments emphasizing its socially constructed nature, only to reappear with vigor as a biological entity in the early twenty-first century.[51] Thus, in terms of racial history as a constructed lens through which to view the past, particularly the gendered past, genomic science offered new truth claims about the prehistory of race.[52]

HeLa exemplifies and Henrietta Lacks personifies the regenerative persistence of this sub-Saharan-African genetic possibility and ability, carrying with it the narrative baggage of the racialized black matriarch. Further illustrating the historical conflation of ancestry with gender, and race with genetics, researchers at the University of California, Berkeley, in 1987 argued for an original mitochondrial ancestor of all humanity. The scientific narrative of the sub-Saharan, Out-of-Africa origins of humanity soon found itself in tension with Judeo-Christian origin narratives based on religious myth. Subsequently interpreted through a gendered Western religious lens, this mitochondrial ancestor, or "genetic matriarch," was envisioned as Eve from the biblical Garden and was sometimes referred to as "Mitochondrial Eve," who in turn became known as "African Eve."[53] Some saw this development as a compromise between science and religion. Others saw it as a simplistic racialization of an extremely complex story of human variation. Analyses of race and gender, imbricated within evolutionary theory, had moved from the "bare bones" of the fossil to gendered explanations of sub-Saharan-African genetic ancestry.[54]

In the above cases, scholarship about human genetic ancestry proved permeable to perennial constructions of race and gender. Empirical sample data, first attributed descriptively through observation, were subsequently ascripted interpretively using categories demarcating inherited social statuses (matriarchal, religious, racial, gender, etc.) and therefrom imbued with explanatory characteristics of hierarchical social value. As social facts, such ascripted statuses are then read scientifically as inherited, not achieved. I base my understanding on earlier anthropological work on ascripted status and the sociology of ascriptive inequality to offer a broader analytic that moves beyond attribution as description to ascription as explanation.[55] As for example, in the British system of *hereditary peerages*, ascription or ascripted status refers to a social standing inherited from birth. By contrast, achieved status refers to merit-based social standing accomplished during one's lifetime, as in the British system of *life peerages*. Women rarely receive peerages, except in the absence of a male heir or by special writ. Except in special cases, the descendants of women peers generally cannot inherit their mother's title or peerage.[56]

Perplexingly therefore, the term *matriarch* used to describe Henrietta Lacks runs counter to anthropological definitions of matriarchy as an intergenerational female right to political and economic power. Matriarchal societies pass on status and wealth to children through the maternal line and, more importantly, women in these societies figure prominently in the total political and economic structure of the group. As anthropologist Peggy Sanday notes, matriarchal societies trace not only temporal but cosmological descent from a female ancestor/progenitor/goddess, thereby sacralizing social practices that legitimate the social order between and among the sexes.[57] Seen this way, matriarchy does not imply the political or economic power to subjugate others but the power to conjugate and regenerate the totality of social life. In contrast, matrifocal (or matricentric) groups are female-headed households characterized in Creole societies by racialized forms of male exclusion from the larger socioeconomic sphere.[58]

Children in matrilineal groups inherit positive status and, often, rights to resources reckoned through the maternal line. Unlike the integral social role matriarchy serves, matrifocality exists within the interstices and at the margins of larger socioeconomic forces. Children in these families inherit neither positive status nor resources (or rights to them) from their mothers.

Other scholars have critiqued matriarchal discourses as self-indulgent practices in status elevation removed from their racialized context. For these scholars, matriarchy as a concept explains precious little while gratuitously describing a nonexistent kinship structure. Matriarchy, as expounded upon by nineteenth-century scholars such as Edward Tylor and twentieth-century scholars such as W. H. R. Rivers, found little support from empirical studies, which thus stated that matriarchy no longer existed. If it ever did, it did so within overarching patriarchal kinship structures either through patrilineal marriage or matrilineal brother/uncle rubrics.[59] Matriarchy assumes inherited female rights to resources and influence in political decision making. Hence, in the Lacks case, the characterization of "matriarch" is curious, given that it finds little to no definitional or objective traction. Worse still, it crowds out conversations about matrifocality as an intergenerational process of gendered dispossession.[60] Yet, it is not enough to simply dismiss Lacks's ascribed status of "matriarch" as a matter of poor word choice, however unintentional. Rather, because it circulates within wider scientific narratives on African origins and genetic "Eves," the usage of *matriarch* exemplifies larger problems around locating research wealth and excavating the material-discursive makings of race and gender.

FINDING METABOLIC AFRICA IN THE ADMIXED MATRIARCH

Scientific discourses about Henrietta Lacks and HeLa cells have long reflected these epistemic, definitional, and methodological issues. When Walter Nelson-Rees received six cell samples from the Soviet Union in 1973, he believed them to have originated in female donors. The cells were all revealed to possess only X-shaped chromosomes, meaning they had the genetic markers for maternal origin and descent. Upon closer examination by Ward Peters in Detroit, all six "Soviet" samples were determined to have originated from a sub-Saharan-African female—to be specific, an "admixed African American" female, Henrietta Lacks.

The publication of the HeLa genome and epigenome in August 2013 was preceded and accompanied by debates about health disparities, genomic explanations for differential disease outcomes among racial groups, and the politics of racial classification and their intersections with power, purity, admixture, and ethnoracial self-identification. However, the dual lives of Henrietta Lacks and the immortal HeLa cell line trouble these health disparity debates, biological discourses on racial purity and Creole admixture, and attendant claims to locate and source sub-Saharan-African genetic diversity in the human genome, figuring what Spillers calls the "undecipherability of black flesh" even in the face of these widespread, organizational attempts to decode it.[61]

Embodying the diversity of sub-Saharan mtDNA in a racially admixed family, the body of Henrietta Lacks revolutionized cellular biology and spurred global biomedical research. The sequencing of the HeLa genome and epigenome in 2013 promised, or threatened, to change the way we understood metabolic adaptation to environmental change, while offering new opportunities to better understand the biological mechanisms involved in Type 2 diabetogenesis. It raised ethical questions about who should profit from that understanding. Race, gender, and ascripted, or inherited, matriarchal social status intertwined within regimes of property ownership and drew a bioethical line between novel forms of exchange and historical regimes of appropriation. Moreover, it accentuated this bioethical line dually with the wealth dynamics of the racial gift as a cultural form of social exchange and the gendered commodity as an item of market exchange.

MATRIARCHAL DISPOSSESSION AND RACIALIZED PARTICIPATION

It is not difficult to source the missing intergenerational wealth implied in the matriarchal designation given to Henrietta Lacks. The HeLa cell line has founded a global research industry that has generated over a half century's worth of professional and scientific capital. A search on the PubMed Central database turns up approximately 138,000 research papers written and nearly 60,000 NIH grants awarded over the last six decades about HeLa and its central role in developing effective vaccines for both poliomyelitis and the human papilloma viruses.[62] Yet, somehow achieving a just calculus of balanced reciprocity among the Lacks family, the scientific community, and the wider society benefiting from HeLa research remained an unformulated equation.

The publishing of the HeLa genome and epigenome prompted media speculation about negotiations between the NIH and the Lacks family concerning the possible payment of royalties to the family. As reported in *Nature,* this presented a dilemma for Francis Collins:

> Some Lacks family members raised the possibility of financial compensation, Collins says. Directly paying the family was not on the table, but he and his advisers tried to think of other ways the family could benefit, such as patenting a genetic test for cancer based on HeLa-cell mutations. But they couldn't think of any.[63]

Although financial compensation was not ultimately granted, two members of the Lacks family were subsequently included on the ethics board charged with formulating the appropriate conditions for obtaining HeLa genome samples for research. Board inclusion was framed as an equitable step toward medical justice, despite the family's deepening intergenerational poverty, relative scientific illiteracy, and sparse social capital—and all of this in fact risked furthering the exploitation that inclusion sought to redress. Johns Hopkins University, moreover, created two scholarship programs in the name of Henrietta Lacks and promised that 40 percent of new hires at the university would come from inner city Baltimore. For the Lacks family, monetary recompense is for the most part generated through speaking appearances and private donations made by those particularly touched by the story of Henrietta Lacks and HeLa.

Henrietta Lacks's birth in the former slave quarters of a Virginia tobacco plantation highlighted the sociogenesis of a racialized social hierarchy that would later relegate her to the colored ward of a hospital in which she sought treatment for cervical cancer, and from which her now immortal cells were harvested. Over sixty years later, her cells continue to replicate in laboratories around the world, persisting alongside questions of ethics, consent, and social justice. And having "contaminated" upward of 20 percent of the cell lines used in research globally, she continues to cross biological boundaries policed by the social order that characterized the world in which she lived and died.

In Chapel Hill, Dr. Mikel couched his excitement about new genomic analytical technologies with a dose of skepticism concerning the stories these technologies cannot tell:

> Genomics cannot determine or predict disease risk, much less the height of an individual, or for that matter, a group. Genetics cannot tell stories outside of history. We need more fully sequenced genomes and exomes from populations with diverse demographic histories. We also need to fully map *past ancestry* before we can confidently predict *future risk*. At this point in time, we can talk about patterns and processes, but can say nothing at all about the people themselves. (author's emphasis)

Dr. Mikel's allusion to history proved interstitial to many of the presentations and conversations in Raleigh-Durham. The meeting, therefore, brought to the surface the uneasy balancing of the *necessity* of African-descent genomic research inclusion and participation in the generation of future knowledge with the bioethics of such inclusion and participation. The bioethical history of Henrietta Lacks's life and HeLa's immortal behavior transgresses the rational boundaries of society and science, labor and expertise, and their constructed social mechanisms of racial inclusion and exclusion. The Lacks case reflects these suspicious histories and constitutes neither accident nor coincidence, nor even malign intent, but rather the genomic fulfillment of long-standing social, economic, and structural processes. It reveals impoverishment structures existing within larger patriarchal wealth accumulation networks and offers an optics for examining kinship in making legible the sociocultural construction of both research recruitment and health disparities. I submit that these biosocial forms of wealth accumulation and status regulation are not acquired through merit but are ascripted by birth within hierarchical gift relations reflecting gendered and raced disparities in both social capital and social justice. Such disparities render elusive ethical notions of informed consent and research equity.

The matriarchal label attached to Henrietta Lacks forecloses a clearer understanding of an "irredeemable past" in which the "present was the future that had been created by men and women in chains, by human commodities, by chattel persons."[64] Sethe, in Toni Morrison's *Beloved,* struggles against such a social order, one built on racialized and commodified reproduction that legitimates acts of bioappropriation based neither on consent nor reciprocity. However, such culturally legitimated acts, based not on the "protected relationships" assumed by Mauss, insist on the right to obligate the giver to gift through participation in asymmetrical forms of exchange.[65] To paraphrase Sanday and DuBois, Sethe refused to conjugate merely to perpetuate and consequentially subjugate her descendants to biological existences conditioned upon reproducing intergenerational obligations to exchange sacrificially as racial labor gifted to the nation. Seen through this prism, I suggest the impossibility of achieving matrifocal justice or assuming matriarchal power to effect the ethical reformation of racialized social practices. I build on the work of Joan Scott in positing that kinship alone does not reproduce gender, but that both gender and race are constituted in large part separately from kinship by political and economic forces operating in the wider society.[66]

REPRODUCING MATRIARCHY, REPRODUCING DIVERSITY

Both anthropology and sociology have contributed mightily to the rise, fall, and genomic resurrection of the empty matriarchal crown. In the twenty-first-century genomic moment, the political economy of race and matriarchy took on new salience in authoring new participatory regimes of wealth accumulation, relying on older, gendered forms of social engagement and obligations to give and receive that legitimated appropriation in the absence of informed consent. The racial body as a diverse, regenerative product of power and history marks mercantile colonial, capitalist industrial, and contemporary biocapital epochs. Authorial power and historical narratives recirculating matriarchal discourses insinuate an elevated kinship status neither ascripted by birth nor achieved through merit. These narratives reproduce the social order, the racial body, and, geographically, the neighborhoods and zip codes demarcating race, gender, socioeconomic status, and disparate health outcomes. This arguably informs the understandings of diverse communities that the original Framingham researchers had urged over sixty years ago.

Dr. Barrington was adamant:

> Genomics and genetics will not narrow health disparities—they may actually increase them. Class, race, and racism are more

reliable indicators of health. However, "race" is a crude proxy for shared biological and environmental backgrounds—yet, there is no way to scientifically tease out the biological from the environmental.

I suggest that the original Framingham researchers did not fully comprehend the ways race, gender, socioeconomic status, and health disparities naturalize through circulating social discourses that make tenuous but durable associations with biology. They did point to a future focus on the epigenetic, or recently acquired biological and environmental variables contributing to what they presciently suspected were differential factors affecting disparate health outcomes in diverse communities. But to repeat, the Framingham researchers did not code difference, disparity, and diversity in racial terms or attribute causation uniquely to them.

The mapping of the genome and epigenome of HeLa offers a microcosmic narrative of constructed race, gender, history, and inequality that traveled metabolically with the seas across the Atlantic. There, its metabolism adapted to the new environment, biologically and socially, laboring under the watchful eye of racial capital, patriarchal surveillance, and the burning sun. One day, sub-Saharan Africa escaped from these shackles, demonstrating a biological persistence, in vivo and in vitro, that could not, however, escape its compromised relationship to privacy, to agency, to society itself. Type 2 diabetes, a significant aspect of this genealogy of racialized adaptation, or better, a genealogy of adaptation to the notion of race, sheds light on the contingent possibilities of eliminating health disparities in the absence of the human dignity that only justice can provide.

The contingent possibilities of eliminating health disparities in the future, therefore, must accompany both a vigilant bioethical memory and vigilant bioethical safeguarding. But who should remember and who should safeguard bioethical vigilance?

As one African-descent researcher related in 2012,

> We should feel responsible for the educating, increasing the
> health literacy of the African American population, and having a
> presence at the table in these discussions about genomic research
> and African American participation in trials. Because of the
> amounts of funding available for race-based health disparities

genomics research, there are people who could care less about the health of minority and poor people who have climbed on the bandwagon. We are the conscience that will ensure the Tuskegees and Guatemalas don't happen again.[67]

Dr. Odu located bioethical responsibility in both African-descent and minority researchers as a frontline collective vanguard against documented amoral bioscientific impulses. Echoing Dr. Ralston's sentiment expressed earlier, Dr. Odu maintained that race-based research on minority bodies predicated on reducing health disparities among racial minorities is not driven by an altruistic bioethics of care. Instead, recruitment and knowledge production in health disparities work is impelled by a pragmatic political economy of inclusion, the research opportunities presented by rapid technological advancement, and the possibilities of robust asset value creation.

The race to detect sugar in the blood and decode racial metabolisms of risk was superseded by more lucrative, technological modes of anticipating and speculating upon its prediagnostic predictive value. The sheer speed of technological and discursive change about diabetes risk from 2008 to 2013 reflected the dynamism of the field and how, as a social scientist, to define it. The unveiling of the DRS in 2008 occurred during the same year genomic sequencing costs began their precipitous downward slide. By 2011, the DRS was well on its way to commercial and clinical irrelevance. Meanwhile, the three-year period from 2008 to 2011 witnessed a decrease in sequencing costs from around US$100,000 to less than $3,000. Enabled by these developments, the genome and epigenome of HeLa was mapped in 2013, the same year Tethys BioSciences began formulating an exit strategy for the DRS. Hiding race within a Type 2 diabetes risk algorithm proved less provocative explanatorily and less evocative historically than the metabolic legacy of Henrietta Lacks and her emblematic representation of Creole history as a relationship to labor and capital that enculturated racial and gendered obligations to give, sacrifice, and submit without guarantee of reciprocal consideration.

I am confident that an approach centering on the gendered intersections of labor and capital would recontextualize both Neel and Framingham in demonstrating the environmental, not racial, contingency of Type 2 diabetes risk. HeLa moves our conversation from the gross flesh and bone of enslaved racial anatomies to the subtler liberatory bioenergetics of mitochondrial persistence and environmental adaptation. In doing so, it inverts patriarchal narratives of racial resilience in ways that Morrison, Spillers, Holloway, Hartman, and other black feminist writers have illustrated—and through which, in their scriptural validation, HeLa actualizes.

REPRODUCING THE BIOECONOMY

Matriarchy, specifically black matriarchy, as a vital yet underexamined contextual analytic in the social and political sciences, encapsulates historical forms of exchange, obligations to participate, and the arbitrary power of reciprocity. Through the case of Henrietta Lacks, the economically (re)productive, commodified, and laboring black female slave reemerged as an economically (re)producing, commodifiable, laboring, status-elevated black matriarch. Neither an accident of racial, gender, or sexual history, nor a coincidence of physiological pathology and reproductive regeneration (or for that matter an exemplar of social deviance), she eventually crossed the segregated lines of kinship, desire, and race to redefine exchange, integration, and contamination in both society and biology.

The political economy of matriarchy undergirding media and scientific narratives around HeLa links to older histories of racial and gendered practices of exchange and appropriation. "She," whether the primordialized "Mitochondrial Eve," racialized "African Eve," or the "admixed" Henrietta Lacks, demonstrates how "she" was rendered fecund and exploitable in bioeconomic knowledge production. Consequently, as an ascripted matriarch having no real ability to effect change in the social order, her descendants live in relative poverty. She and most black "matriarchs" in the United States struggle against a downward intergenerational spiral of health and economic disparities, kinship instability, and their disparate intersections with social, economic, and medical justice. Further, she and her descendants indict what Annemarie Mol calls "the logic of care" to expose its illogicality by simply asking, "What has the category done for me?"[68]

The bioethics of black matriarchy highlights the analytical importance of examining discourses that valorize sacrificial exchange and the elevated status claims ascripted to the obligated. Coveting the bioenergetics that animate bodies guarantees little in terms of social justice for those bodies embedded in at-risk families, communities, and populations. It is this critique that finds changes in the Common Rule inadequate. Examining redesigned efforts toward achieving social justice and eliminating health disparities via programmatic mechanisms of inclusion and consent requires making robust analytical distinctions between the sacrificial inequality of participation and the bioethics of appropriation, along the axes of power they inhabit. The future will determine whether the true bioethical value of gift recruitment can facilitate balanced reciprocity commensurate to the imagined biovalue of race and gender.

Conclusion

The Racialized Pancreas

TOWARD BIOSOCIAL JUSTICE

> Starting with the deliberately chosen example of the most
> artificial normalization, technological normalization, we can
> grasp an invariable characteristic of normality. Norms are
> relative to each other in a system, at least potentially. Their
> co-relativity within a social system tends to make this system
> an organization, that is, a unity in itself, if not by itself and
> for itself.
>
> —Georges Canguilhem, *On the Normal and the Pathological*

This book presents three case studies in which science, technology, and medicine emerged with new race-based recruitment strategies based upon racially differentiated disease profiles. The ethnographic snapshots I had taken chronicled rapid changes in the science and technology of Type 2 diabetes. They signal a speculative movement toward technologies of risk and away from technologies of diagnosis.

Georges Canguilhem framed a phenomenological context in which the artificial could be rendered normal through a social system of organized technological practices. I have attempted to show that biological "norms" as well as "risks" share co-relativity within wider political and economic systems of sociocultural relations. I stop short, however, of fully locating the "deliberately chosen example of the most artificial normalization" in technology itself.[1] I argue that the most artificial normality begins with the concept of biological race, not only as a measurable norm but also as a measurable risk. Genetic and genomic research cannot locate race as a bioassessment; short of this, racial biomarkers for Type 2 diabetes remain elusive.

The Age of Discovery, the Enlightenment, the Industrial Revolution, and the concomitant rise of science heralded a historical trajectory of durable metabolic significance. These moments facilitated the industrialization of both scientific knowledge and sugar production, and their global diffusion. In other words, science and sugar, as racial projects, created new categories of human difference in relationship to labor, capital, and production. Even in areas of the world that did not participate in sugar production, sweeteners hidden in foods have begun to elicit concern about their contribution to the prevalence of obesity, Type 2 diabetes, and the burdens they pose upon public health and clinical health care systems. Earlier antislavery abolitionist admonitions that sugar was stained with blood yielded to a twentieth-century search for blood stained with sugar. In the twenty-first century the search has begun for inherent ancestral vulnerabilities to the stain of sweetness itself. These three moments attest to the enduring utility, profitability, and tractability of black bodies as sacrificial indexes of progress. Nevertheless, with an increasingly sedentary global cross-section of humanity wading in a pool of excess calories, racial theories of diabetes risk persist, despite evidence of our diversely shared metabolic contributions toward the obesity and Type 2 diabetes epidemics and the creation of a Type 2 diabetes industry.

In the West, the age of production ushered in a subsequent age of consumption. Consequently, bodily practices forged by and fueled for production have, for the most part, been replaced by global bodies slackened by consumption and new forms of technosocialized inertia. New technological tools can now measure the metabolic effects of this historical shift from productive labor to consumptive labor. As this book has shown, these tools and techniques introduce and operationalize new pharmaceutical entrées for treating Type 2 diabetes, prediabetes, and diabetes risk itself within the contexts of people's lives.

In the case of Tethys's Diabetes Risk Score (DRS) technology, its authorial representatives proffered a truth claim about a new technological form of predictive veridiction. However, genetic and genomic discourses of disease occurrence pushed the risk-predictive authority of science even further back in time in ways that may make diabetes risk algorithms such as the DRS and even the glucometer obsolete. The amount of funding pouring into genetic and genomic research dwarfs whatever private capital Tethys BioSciences could have ever reasonably hoped to attract. Media, scientific, and other institutional actors constantly circulate conversations about genetics and genomics. These conversations saturate social life. While it can be argued whether genetic and genomic discourses rebiologize notions of race,

I argue that these discourses do inevitably rebiologize notions of difference. Given this discursive power, in ways possibly more persuasive than the DRS, genetic and genomic articulations of risk based on difference may in the future convey not the possibility of risk, but a confirmation of diagnosis as a social fact. As a form of personalized medicine, genomic difference as individualized risk could come to supplant race as group risk, but not racially supplant the individual categorically.

The future development of genomic target drugs to treat risk based on genomic difference could conceivably do away with the social inconveniences of current diet, lifestyle, and pharmaceutical approaches to managing diabetes. Such drugs, so defined, would perhaps shift the language from that of diabetes management to one of diabetes prophylaxis. However promising new genetic and genomic research into disease causation and health disparities may be, no new reliable biomarkers have emerged from these investigations. At this point in time, neither race nor genomics offers global guidance or clear instruction for improving medical outcomes. Moreover, genetic and genomic investigations leading to declarations of links between ancestry, ascribed race, and Type 2 diabetes remain both tenuous and premature. Genome-disease associations have yet to generate firm correlations that would confidently transform susceptibility into risk, and even further down the line, any bioassessment of risk that would qualify for candidacy as an eventual diagnostic biomarker. A bioassessment is not a biomarker, and a biomarker is not a disease. Nonetheless, or perhaps due to these incongruences, the genetic diversity of African-descent and comparatively othered populations are seen as bankable biocurrency on the thoroughfare to future scientific discovery. Tantalizingly, the biovalue inhered to the genetic diversity of African-descent populations offers researchers many biological variables to explore.

Narrative truth claims couched in the language of association, correlation, and causation may construct a model of a Type 2 pathological gun, even a smoking gun, but have yet to explain the trigger mechanism that prompts such a gun to fire. I question whether biogenetic risk as an estimable, predictive categorical construction of epidemiological inevitability can be neatly superimposed racially onto disparate social landscapes and divergent diasporas. As the Tethys, Mt. Zion, and biopharma/genomics examples show, risk discourse, policy, and participant aversion are highly dependent upon class, educational attainment, and subjective positionalities within the fields of power of any given society.[2]

REIMAGINING EXPERTISE

I point to the translational challenges facing biotechnological, clinical, and bench scientific research in effectively accessing, communicating with, and recruiting at-risk target populations. In effect, I argue that health disparities often begin at the top, based on incomplete knowledge of the cultural, economic, and social factors animating targeted population groups, as well as their historical construction, all of which inform their real health care needs. Expanding the ranks of certified diabetes educators (CDEs) to include community health workers (CHWs), professionals, and others with strong links to their own communities would do much to improve diabetes education outreach efforts. This would ensure that, for example, diabetes walks are not scheduled on Sunday mornings if one wishes to attract large numbers of African Americans—particularly when the institutional imagination envisions African American churches as indispensable to these efforts. However, the relative absence of cultural competence and access to basic health care renders social justice incomplete and distrust in bioscientific research participation rational.

As related in chapter 4, I received enthusiastic support from African American Type 2 diabetes patients, health care professionals, and researchers who cited the need for more African American research expertise concerning the illness. While I was mildly surprised by the exhortations from the lay community, those from African American health care professionals came rather unexpectedly. What both groups explicitly suggested is the importance of African American researchers' involvement in the bioethical generation of scientific knowledge production. As in the case of Tuskegee, "knowledge" produced by a group with high social capital about a group with low social capital should be seen and studied through the bioethical research lenses of the group over and under study. Tuskegee, the DRS, and now genomic science hold out African-descent groups and comparative others as desirable population samples that will increase the power of the instruments that researchers hope will one day become clinical tools. What remains unclear is whether these tools will help fashion future biosocial justice. The past and the present offer no sources of effusive optimism, especially since the social determinants of health filter infusively and diffusively through the genetic research and the biomedical industrial complexes.

I have aimed to show that cultural competence primarily addresses bounded ethnic and racial categories instead of complex, nuanced community contexts. Rochester, like many areas of the world, illustrates that neighborhoods, communities, diasporas, and ethnoracial categories have different, sometimes overlapping boundaries and forms of boundary making. Some categorical boundaries, such as *race* and *ethnicity, community* and *neighborhood,* or *expert* and *expertise,* have no discrete edges. Bounded by their own descriptors, citizen-subjects become proxied boundary-objects used in everyday biopolitical language and practice.[3]

Further, Type 2 diabetes is an epidemiological, social, and economic phenomenon that, I cannot help but aver, intricately demonstrates how use-cum-exchange values subordinate and subsume social relations. Public health prompts to get tested, media prompts to obtain free and discounted glucometers, and urgings of prediabetics (as members of a new illness category) to self-test raise important questions concerning how affect is produced through technological (self)-inculcation. (Self)-experimentation restructures knowledges and further problematizes existence. The development of the genetic ancestry market further complicates epistemological and ontological knowledge structures and narratives of existence and belonging.[4]

I have attempted to help fill an ethnographic void by highlighting how scientists, clinicians, public health professionals, and venture capitalists reconfigure their practices to the specificities of changing subjects, objects, and milieux in contesting and reproducing the scientific autonarrative of racial risk.[5] Therefore, this research has sought to address the ways in which diabetes has been recast as a technology of quantitative risk informing patient behavior and agency. It illustrates the roles of industry, scientific, and medical-consumer networks in redefining not only the illness but also recruitment along the ascripted categories of *patient, consumer,* and *citizen.*

A NEW BIOECONOMIC MOMENT

The precarious economic climate at the end of the first and beginning of the second decades of the twenty-first century made venture capitalists more risk averse and consequently less patient with bio-technology firms' five- and seven-year proposed research-to-market timelines. Yet given the amount of money funneled into research over the last four decades, increasing pressure has been placed on bio-technological research in light of the disappointing record of generating improved health and financial outcomes in hollowing out the current research Valley of Death. I situated this discussion and larger research agenda within a new Type 2 diabetes technological moment: the temporal shift in the clinical gaze from *diagnostic* to *predictive* accuracy and from *illness* to *risk*, respectively. Ultimately, this temporal shift makes us question whether public health outreach can successfully overcome the strategic corporate ideologies and innovative technological advances responsible for the sedentary construction of the contemporary Type 2 diabetic subject—or, if such a possibility runs counter to the fundamental ethos and interests of the market itself.

I questioned throughout my research how contemporary diabetes risk organizes and frames these public health and bioclinical recruitment strategies and allied discourses. I examined how the cultural, epidemiological, and social attention shifts from the event (or the disease) to the risk of the event occurring, contributing to the enrollment of new actors in new roles under new labels of consumer, citizen, patient, subject. The Framingham Study signaled the need for diversity inclusion in future cardiometabolic research, while ironically describing the ideal socioeconomic rationales for its original research-recruitment strategy. The subsequent ADVANCE, ACCORD, DPP, and VADT trials demonstrated the limits of pharmaceutical blood-glucose control methods in the absence of a comprehensive approach that addresses the overall cardiometabolic life of the patient.

Fieldwork led me to conclude that Type 2 diabetes technologies may suggest rational biopharmaceutical interventions. However, patient subjectivity carries its own rationalities that neither the market nor the clinic can predict or rely upon. Of significance here is that what remains central to the unanticipated emergence of Type 2 diabetes subjectivities is the technology itself. The glucometer, OGTT, HbA1c test, or for that matter, the DRS, in the end can only serve as a call to action, to practice. Yet these prophylactic and therapeutic actions or practices do not always unfold in the biopolitical spaces of communities imagined in the clinical, public health, or biomarket spaces of the biotech and pharmaceutical industries—nor are they always informed by them. Technologies of control are not necessarily controlling technologies.

African Americans, in Tethys's view, represented a racial/ethnic group with discrete, definable, and translatable boundaries that could be operationalized in a clinical trial. However, defining their target market racially threatened to limit the applicability of the technology to specific nations. The innovative clinical and market challenges facing Tethys revolved around developing a precision instrument that could find global applicability across a broad spectrum of different biopolitical categories of race/ethnicity and different bioeconomic regimes of value.

I suggest that making race, risk, and the future fungible, or interchangeable, as both a knowledge demand and form of capital logic, constituted the biosocial amalgam rendered invisible within DRS technology. This technologically embedded racial invisibility creates room for interpretive ambiguity: Separating facts from both subjective interpretations of difference and market discourses of value problematizes what is truly worth knowing about Type 2 diabetes and the racialized body—particularly when the subject has, herself, been subsumed within the science and rendered invisible, racially, within the technology. Race and risk as social facts circulate discursively, politically, and scientifically, but do not necessarily morally constrain the individual to adhere to or comply with prescribed diabetes regimens, despite the cardiometabolic punishment, in a Durkheimian sense, that deviance guarantees.

This book has engaged the ways that race, as a most artificial normality, continues to operate with contingent success within a social system of organized scientific and economic practices. The concept of bioethical matriarchy highlights the analytical importance of examining raced and gendered discourses that valorize sacrificial exchange and the elevated status claims ascripted to the obligated. Justice demands unrelenting and unwavering attention to the ways discourses of race and gender continue to operate productively within a social system of organized scientific and economic practices involved in the perennial deciphering of black flesh. In this social system of organized practices, race as epidemiological risk and gender as inherited risk become mobilized in creating new forms of economic reward. Translating risk into reward presents yet another definition of the Valley of Death, but not necessarily its solution.

TRANSCENDING INCLUSION

Examining efforts toward achieving social justice via programmatic mechanisms of inclusion and consent requires making robust distinctions between the sacrificial inequality of participation and the bioethics of appropriation, along the axes of power they inhabit. The future will determine whether the true bioethical value of the gift can facilitate balanced reciprocity commensurate to the imagined biovalue of race and gender.[6] Nevertheless, the consumer-citizen, enrolled in a lifelong climb up a steep learning curve, is seen as a privatized manager of biological risk for public health and biomedical institutions as well as a plethora of data points of biovalue for biotech and clinical research stakeholders.[7] Citizenship is a technology of different forms of government requiring different forms of discipline *in relation to others*.[8] "Give me your body and I will give you meaning. I will make you a name and a word in my discourse."[9] Racial and behavioral categories provide room for new explanations of risk, disease, and care for different populations in relation to each other. As social beings claiming and embodying multiple identities, the consumer-citizen-patient, through relational obligations, labors in new ways.[10]

In the nineteenth and most of the twentieth centuries, care of the self as both personal and medical practice existed relationally in terms of social and biological conformity, of the norm. Advances in genetic, genomic, and postgenomic research in the late twentieth and early twenty-first centuries have shaped a new personalized medicine based not on sociobiological conformity but on genetic diversity and individual biological uniqueness. While this book has sought to highlight the biosocial tension between diversity and homogeneity, I reaffirm Du Bois that both reinscribe kinship hierarchies through the new and perennial narratives they author.

Kinship in the form of genomic risk associations also calls into question epidemiological understandings of population health, as precision medicine's future stakes depend on the development of economically attractive and technologically precise genomic assessments of individual disease risk. However, the pharmaceutical industry would have to contend with an epistemic and methodological shift in focus from *demos* to *ego*. Pharmaceutical profitability has long been rooted in the development of blockbuster drugs and, as a former biotechnology executive stated, "repeat users."[11] One alternative strategy would use genetic truth claims to target "the worried well," bringing an increased emphasis on the immeasurable subjectivity of "wellness" instead of the measurable objectivity (and accounting) of "health."[12]

The production of blockbuster drug profitability predicates itself on the epidemiology and biostatistics of population health. That said, pharmaceutical concerns would have to grapple with a promised precision medicine rooted in individually determined genomic risk factors dependent upon the generation of massive data sets obtained from grouped populations, communities, and families. In the meantime, research continues apace, exploring genomic causes of obesity and Type 2 diabetes—as well as drugs aimed at their control. I have attempted to situate the research recruitment of people of African descent within an ethnographic history of diabetes, its earlier and contemporary racialized framings, and the instruments and technologies employed in translating, reinterpreting, and redefining the illness along collapsed temporal lines of clinical interpretation.

This book engaged the shifting illness metaphors and signifiers that Type 2 diabetes represents, the speculative discourses of risk they circulate, and the possibilities for a certain form of contemporary self-care within the habitus of truth that this particular Type 2 diabetes technological moment imparts. A concomitant rise in human inertia has enabled this epochal shift in technological engagement with "blood sugar." The way we live now has witnessed its biological predicate in the increased prevalence in obesity and Type 2 diabetes. Technology not only enabled this shift: it measures, indexes, monitors, and surveys its movement in a digitized effort to help us chart our individual and collective metabolic demise.

However, as dual ideological products of society and the market, both technology and Type 2 diabetes each contain agentic possibilities that can challenge hegemonic discourses of risk and race. In other words, racial narratives of risk allow contingent room to envision a certain kind of life, a certain kind of freedom, a certain kind of knowing as a truth-seeking subject. This book gestures toward a transcendent subject who exists within the margins as a statistical outlier in the midst of ethnoracial discourses, metaphors, ironies, technologies, programs, and facts concerning pathological sweetness—a cultivator of a certain kind of authenticity in an increasingly designed and engineered world. This prescribes ethnographic, historical, and other forms of qualitative research to explicate the statistical outlier as anthropological rule rather than ethnological exception.[13]

Sweetness in the Blood is, in effect, an ethnographic dialogue between self and solution to a racially, historically, and technologically defined and socially interpreted problem: contemporary Type 2 diabetes risk. I wanted to shed vital light on the programmatic practices it rationalizes, the actors it categorizes and seeks to enroll, and the future-oriented relationship between risk, prognosis, and speculation. It is at these intersections of risk, prognosis, and speculation where epistemic battles occur over what is "mere marketing" and what is "pure knowledge."[14]

TRANSLATING FUTURES PAST

An interactive relationship between biology and race exists dichotomously between researchers, a relationship not easily translated.[15] For example, although the mission of the Clinical Research Center (CRC) aims to enroll diabetes and other cardiometabolic patients in pharmaceutical trials, Dr. Asela has uncertain hope that through public outreach in the way of diabetes education classes he might eventually attract African American volunteers. Urban renewal programs in the early 1970s, the decentralization of Rochester to the suburbs, and the demise of the Eastman Kodak Company in the 1980s until the present, as well as gentrification in the 1990s and 2000s, have left Dr. Asela searching for the key that will unlock the door to a hard-to-penetrate African American community. Through this lens the viability and even existence of the social as an imagined public health target must be questioned in translating rational clinical science within "irrationalized zones of human existence."[16] In the meantime, Mt. Zion Baptist Church has taken as its charge the responsibility of community health outreach and service to those irrationalized "zones of social abandonment" within "minoritized spaces," zones of human existence with their own rationalities. These rationalities voice a coherent language Mt. Zion understands quite well based on kinship, shared experiences, and historical discourses about the body, race, community, and biomedicine.[17]

Late nineteenth- and twentieth-century functionalist descriptions of the role of the black church were emblematic of the theoretical conventions of that period. However, I extended this historical lens to focus on contemporary questions about why, where, and under what conditions the church intersected with various biomedical efforts to garner African American research interest and participation. I departed the field convinced that outreach through churches misses at-risk youth and young-adult populations. Fieldwork in Southwest Rochester and at the CRC elicited no contacts with Type 2 diabetics under forty years of age.

Nevertheless, health professional and community stakeholders from diverse backgrounds like Dr. Asela, Robert Mann, Dr. Johnson, and Merlene Bailey are engaged in ongoing translational mediation between science and society. Cultivating trust in a community involves embracing that community's world view and sense of being in the world. As historical witnesses and biomedical subjects, African Americans have had reason to believe that their *experiences*—often reframed as *perceptions* in the descriptive and explanatory language of objective scientific truth and recycled as pastoral care—should arouse *healthy* skepticism. On the other hand, such collective skepticism, what Ruha Benjamin termed "organized ambivalence," may also inform delayed engagement with the health care system while increasing reliance on family and other social-trust networks such as churches, ultimately deepening disparities in terms of timely access to available resources and consequential health outcomes.[18] Yet the Tuskegee Syphilis Study and other significant but lesser-known events serve as cautionary examples of the forms of manipulation that cultural competence can make possible.

The persistence of race-based science requires an anthropological critique beyond the modernity narrative within which it couches itself. Talal Asad reminds that both the anthropological encounter and ethnographic artifact are products of unequal power relationships between the West and the Rest occurring since the emergence of bourgeois Europe, of which colonialism is but one historical moment. Knowledge generated about dominated Others produces "universal understanding" on one hand; on the other, as this book has shown, this knowledge reproduces inequalities in capacity between the Euro-American world and the non-Euro-American world.[19]

Access to the field—as both ethnographic and scientific methods of objectification, as knowledge—has the potential to reify exploitation, as power supports research. In this vital respect, the social and biological sciences walk a fine line between confirming the worlds of the powerful and producing radically subversive forms of understanding these worlds. Asad locates this anthropological "understanding" of world power as a rationality embedded within European languages as discursive products of historically perceiving the world. While anthropology frowns upon those practitioners who "go native," Asad wonders why so few actually have. Intimacy and rapport within the field is mysteriously unproductive in this regard. This asymmetry Asad calls a "dialectic of world power"—anthropological claims of intellectual contribution to understanding are, in the end, subsequent to the structured interests of power, national or corporate. These intellectual works are of more critical importance to the continued receipt of patronage than the interests of power itself. Power affects both theoretical choice and manner of objectifying the field. It is of no surprise, therefore, that the colonial system itself remained unstudied by anthropologists.[20]

Asad makes these points, not to decry anthropology's links to colonialism or its ideological frameworks, but to suggest that as a form of bourgeois consciousness, it contains its own ambiguities and contradictions. These ambiguities and contradictions contain the potentialities of their own transcendence: Anthropology must examine the historical power asymmetries between the North and the South and how as a dialectic they inform the practical conditions of the field, and the epistemic assumptions and multidisciplinary intellectual oeuvres said to represent European understandings of the Other.[21] This project is problematic, as one of these contradictions is that "ever since the Renaissance, the West has sought both to subordinate and devalue other societies, and at the same time to find in them clues to its own humanity."[22]

I agree with Michel-Rolph Trouillot that the modernity narrative invites a question of secondary importance, if only for its heuristic value. Of primary concern are the ways the narrative of modernity works to re-create North Atlantic exceptionalism as the unmarked universal, legitimated through the processes of global capital, and for our purpose, rationalized through the scientific method. Earlier chapters discussed the ways North Atlantic exceptionalism was seen by researchers as too exceptional—a limited biological resource of unconvincingly homogeneous biovalue. Moving forward, more scholarly attention should examine how bioracial geographies are imagined and managed both by capital and triumphalist narratives of Western exceptionalism and normativity.[23] As with the racialized thrifty gene, I submit that this poses important disciplinary questions for the social sciences concerning heterogeneity versus homogeneity as social, political, economic, and academic constructs preventing anthropology from fully emerging from the othered shadows of ethnology.

BIOVALUE GENERATION TOWARD BIOSOCIAL JUSTICE

Attempts at creating future market value through speculation in the bioeconomy depend in part on a cogent and coherent articulation of future clinical value. The case of the PreDx™ DRS represented a technologically enabled shift in the continuing redefinition of diagnosis and the pharmaceutical turn toward medicating risk. From protodiabetes to prediabetes, to diabetic risk prediction, what exactly constitutes *prediabetes* continues to move further backward in physiological time toward mitochondrial Africa. Both homogeneity and diversity served as methodological metaphors for race in developing a more precise biotechnological instrument. Yet race as a conceptual rubric did not function predictably as biology or as a recruitment project toward a community mobilized successfully.

Tethys BioSciences saw its attempts to test its PreDx™ DRS and increase its market and clinical validity as predicated upon outreach to a population-dense yet strategically unknown African American community. The company hoped through public outreach to attract African Americans into its DRS research platform. Tethys thought a sociopolitically constructed racial category valuable in the production of a risk-prediction tool of which race was not used explicitly as an operational variable. It sought to build race into the instrument itself. Collapsing older sociopolitical constructs of group difference, such as race and ethnicity, with more recent biological mappings of phenotype, genotype, and so forth combined with the mathematical rationalities provided by the PreDx™ DRS algorithm offered new interpretive schemata for Type 2 diabetes claim making. Tethys faced significant market hurdles in generating asset value from the DRS, as well as subsequent clinical pushback about the scientific accuracy and practical relevance of the technology within the time constraints of its venture capital funding. The inherent ambiguities of anticipating future profit through calculated illness risk embraces the speculative rationale of the biotechnological market. As shared in chapter 4, the market embraces, if somewhat uneasily and always provisionally, the predictive and diagnostic ambiguities inherent to these technologies, their interpretive frameworks, and frameworkers.

Bioscientific inclusion without social inclusion will remain a problematic and illusive goal as long as an asymmetrical relationship exists between biocapital and social justice. The situation in Rochester and Baltimore reminds us of the ongoing irony surrounding the existence of health care disparities occurring most often in areas adjacent to world-class medical universities and teaching hospitals.[24] Research inclusion within political and epidemiological categories seems to guarantee little with respect to effective therapeutic inclusion. Making sense of the medical implies a multiplicity of flexible subjectivities and learning styles.[25]

African Americans, Native Americans, Latinos, women, prisoners, and military personnel (among others) have accrued biological research value over the course of medical and biotechnological history. The urging of the original Framingham scientists to expand cardiometabolic research efforts to other U.S. subpopulations beyond an all-white community in New England implicated spatial segregation as a social incubator of unknown research value: Tuskegee exploited the spatial and social isolation, as well as the demographic concentration, of its relatively homogeneous target research population. Conversely, research value, premised originally on examining the ravages of Type 2 diabetes in a Native American community living in relative geographic isolation, took an unethical turn by using tribal blood samples to examine biological resilience, human adaptation, and inbreeding. Rochester's Third and Seventh Wards served as the segregated residential geographic boundaries of an African American community devoid today of supermarkets. In the aftermath of racial segregation, urban rebellions, and corporate downturns, diminishing neighborhood options for accessing food exemplify, to paraphrase Ashanté M. Reese, the collision of history and the present in reshaping the precarities of everyday life.[26]

These social, political, and bioeconomic spaces call attention to unequal power arrangements among and between researchers and researched in formulating new narratives of human difference and disease risk. I argue that bioethical scholarship must engage in critical "second-order observation," meaning "observing observers observe" not only of the researchers themselves but also those working in public health, clinical medicine, private practice, as well as in communities.[27] The complicity of researchers and interlocutors of color dating back to Tuskegee rationalizes this approach. This would provide a more robust tracking of how the discursive circulation of power reconfigures the political economy of scientific difference making and subsequent knowledge production—and how these are communicated to at-risk groups. A methodological emphasis that subsumes ethics within an overall focus on justice would bring accompanying analytical rigor toward examining the social and economic politics of consent, inclusion, and participation in bioscientific research. From the standpoint of social justice, the failure to reciprocate to the donor defines Mauss's notion of sacrificial exchange.[28] The challenge of modernity, Mauss argues, is to transform the economy of human relationships from one based on sacrificial exchange to one based on balanced reciprocity.[29] In the case of the HeLa cell line, its perpetual self-laboring, recent genomic and epigenomic sequencing, and discursive accession to matriarchal status and wealth are as ascripted economically as they are intergenerationally.

This necessary widening gaze from the fragmentary biospecimen to the whole person now leaves us several important questions to consider: As a politics of reparation, should a framework for redress prescribe reparative or restorative justice? In other words, can restorative justice make the bioethical matriarch "whole" in a legal sense? Or, can reparative justice render the bioethical matriarch "whole" in an economic sense? And what is more "just": to "repair" and/or to "restore?" These abstract yet vital questions expose the perennial sociocultural dynamics of sacrificial exchange and the failure, inability, or sheer unwillingness to reciprocate.

DELINKING RACE AND TECHNOLOGY

Max Weber advocated understanding technology separately from materialist history and analyses of property relations.[30] The previous chapters of this book suggest otherwise. In regenerating and thereby naturalizing the social order as a social fact, the historical durability of social, biosexual, and scientific modes of reproducing race carry greater socioeconomic value than kinship, which, when emptied of meaningful social content, "can be invaded at any given and arbitrary moment by the property relations."[31] African pan-Americans have been historically commodified as legal property, objectified economically as alienated racial labor, and mined biologically as a natural resource. Property, labor, and resources as gift objects serve as "marker(s) in the economy of human relationships," highlighting specific sociohistorical bonds in which the failure to reciprocate, as with the example of the NIH's treatment of the Lacks family, precedes any legal enforcement or moral or ethical sanction.[32]

Successful outreach efforts demand effective translation and explanation of the variables involved and the stakes concerned. The examples of Tethys BioSciences, the Clinical Research Center, and before in the case of Tuskegee, as well as Henrietta Lacks's family since her death, exemplify a long line of anonymous Others. Recruitment continues apace of a wider community of individuals with neither equitable access to nor resources for obtaining adequate health care.[33] These recruitment efforts continue on the promise of improved future health based on a teleological narrative of biomedical progress and social justice. Yet, make no mistake, this is both a public sector biopolitical and private sector biocapital science of the living and the dead, a dual *vivopolitics* and *necropolitics* of racial biovalue.[34] New-generation genomic sequencing technologies make visible genotypically diverse sub-Saharan *Africanicity* within phenotypically diverse Creole populations, reminding us of the ways alienated labor, capital, and race preconditioned the terms of asymmetrical exchange, biological appropriation, and arbitrary reciprocity over the last 525 years. The gynecological focus of Marion Sims, the hematological focus of Tuskegee, the cytological focus represented by Henrietta Lacks's HeLa cell line, and today, the genealogical focus of contemporary genomics emblematically thread together the historical demand for African-descent bodies and their fragments in scientific research over the last two centuries.[35]

In the United States, previous biomedical research forays into enslaved African bodies marked the nascent chronicling of a necessary bioethical genealogy linking social justice with medical justice punctuating successive slavery, Jim Crow, and post–civil rights movement eras. Diasporic Africa spanned these epochs, contributing a shadow narrative of infusive assimilation into African American society and its racial categories, a narrative that inherently contests territorial definitions of biology and the nation. This bioethical genealogy of racialized research chronologizes different strategies of both overtly and covertly (as well as formally and informally) targeting outreach and translation to this imagined population along a continuum of freedom of choice and moral duty. Framingham, the Danish Inter99 Study, GWAS, Tethys Biosciences, and diversity science highlight different moments of research desire to expand research platforms beyond a limited preponderance of Euro-American data. Such targeted strategies of racial outreach misrecognize the social metabolism of a group as a, using Anthony Hatch's term, "racial metabolism," despite the social, political, and historical constructions of the racial category and its segregated occupants, legatees of bioeconomic engines of inequality and resultant disparity.

Sweetness in the Blood shows the ways technoscientific tools and their promissory rhetorics reconfigure contemporary understandings of Type 2 diabetes within a diagnostic continuum that indexes risk, race, and disease. Type 2 diabetes risk and, for that matter, science and technology know no discrete racial, ethnic, national, or state boundaries, no exclusive temporal or spatial domains. Analytically delinking race from technology, and both from political economy, successfully depends in large part on correcting the error that race, risk, and biology are synonymous, and in this error such belief perpetuates an enduring violence of hope.

THE RACIALIZED PANCREAS AND THE ENDURING VIOLENCE OF HOPE

Betty Washington, the diabetes coordinator at the Alameda Department of Public Health, surmised, "I sometimes wonder about what my pancreas has left, what it can do on its own. I take medication to control my blood sugar levels, exercise when I can, but in the back of my mind, I ask myself if it [the pancreas] can be made healthier, if there is something, an intelligence, that we're not paying attention to." Underlining the market and biosocial relationships presented in this book is the political/economic credibility of racial science as the rational organization of hope. By mediating action in the present, hope controls the emotional levers affecting future senses of the possible. In this way, the body/mind encodes what society says is real.[36] But after all of this classifying, encoding, and translating, how does a racialized organ speak? Can the organ speak?[37]

After all, different speech styles represent and elicit different hope styles. Diagnostic technologies claim to speak for what the organ can and cannot do, or rather, what has happened to the organ—in our case, the pancreas. Glucometers purport to speak for what the organ is doing or has done recently. Diabetes risk scores claim to speak for a pancreas that has not yet contemplated pathological action. Public health understandings and outreach efforts speak using translated interpretations of a racialized pancreas recruited and indexed by risk. Pharmaceuticals claim that they can make the organ speak the true and authentic language of functional normalcy and rational efficiency.

But can pharmaceutical interventions make the racialized pancreas speak, to borrow from John Jackson, *sincerely, authentically*?[38] For that matter, does bariatric surgery answer deeper questions posed by a racialized pancreas in search of the metaphorical sweetness of justice? And if race has no biological basis in fact, can the organ transcend its racially ascribed status? Diet, exercise, and lifestyle arguably articulate no racial claims beyond what not only the organ but indeed the entire cardiometabolic system itself conveys as a result of automediation, of self-agency—which, notably, are the only endogenous forms of bodily mediation related within this paragraph. More radically, can it be said that the pancreas, a pancreas, the pancreas of a Type 2 diabetes patient, has its own narrative of hope, a narrative of organic persistence that bespeaks its own integrity within a bodily constellation of systems, of life processes?

To answer these questions—unsatisfactorily for some—yes and no. Jackson's notion of authenticity depends on an object-subject relationship that reifies the *Othered* subject, much like Gayatri Spivak's subaltern, and in our case, the racialized pancreas.[39] Sincerity, on the other hand, refers to a subject-subject relationship rooted in a common humanity within and between both parties.[40] In this respect, the racialized pancreas can only hope for therapeutic progress through its ongoing objectification. Subsequently, the social determinants driving its racialization get refracted through genetic lenses and treated consequently in and through a myriad of national biopolitical systems and global bioeconomic networks. The social, political, and market terrains this book traverses leads to the speculative promise of the genome and the actualized promise of "personalized medicine." Personalized medicine offers the hope that somewhere down the line an illness is waiting, not necessarily to be cured, but to be prevented. "Hype" keeps that hope alive. Yet hype is far from empty rhetoric, but rather "constitutes the discursive grounds on which reality enfolds."[41] Attaining both wealth and wellness requires conveying speculative cogency in the narrative present.

It is perhaps easier to hope for, to expect, therapeutic change and improvement through pharmaceutical innovation, rather than therapeutic change and improvement through individual and social change. But the net effect of a scientific narrative of hope in the absence of social justice would manifest disparities both old and new, with new and old technological faces and recruited pancreases, speaking new languages generating new hope styles. I argue that violence is embedded within any narrative of progress, particularly scientific narratives, of which this book has highlighted the racial rationalization of health disparities as but one. The historical violence of racial science continues in the face of both natural and social scientific declarations that race as a biological construct has no basis in scientific fact.[42] As this book has amply illustrated, race, unlike neighborhoods, offers no discrete or reliable prediction of biological behavior. And therein lies the violence of claims seeking to link race and risk within unequal narratives of hope.

I present this exposition on violence to focus intently on how social subjects as racial objects become ideologically embedded in new research technologies of risk. As desired research participants, Black Lives do indeed Matter. This book engages the ways in which attempts to evaluate, frame, and put into discursive circulation racialized interpellations of Type 2 diabetes risk were contested or taken for granted, with varying degrees of success. I suggest that inherent limits and intractable dissonances result inevitably from poorly translated attempts to explain how the body, the categorically defined racial body, is inhabited—and addressed.

Acknowledgments

This book is a product of over a decade of collaborative engagement both outside and inside the academy walls. Outside the academy, I thank my San Francisco Bay Area contacts at the Alameda County Department of Public Health, Silicon Valley, and the University of California, San Francisco. In New York, I extend my gratitude to the American Diabetes Association, Mt. Zion Baptist Church, and the Clinical Research Center. I would especially like to thank the entire Rochester community for their interest in my work, and for their efforts to reduce health disparities in the area.

Inside the academy, I especially want to express my profound gratitude to Charis Thompson, Troy Duster, Dána-Ain Davis, and Michel Laguerre. Since this project began, I have benefited greatly from their wise counsel and exemplary collegiality. I hope this book reflects the best of our exchanges. Fatimah Jackson and Lovell Alan Jones provided excellent networking and fieldwork opportunities in North Carolina and Texas, respectively. Their indispensable efforts made it possible to broaden my understanding of health disparities and the recruitment of African-descent populations, as well as the historical and contemporary relationships between historically black colleges and universities, predominantly white institutions, and government health and bioscientific institutions.

A University of California President's Postdoctoral Fellowship in the Department of Sociology at UC Santa Cruz from 2013 to 2015 introduced me to an outstanding department with a remarkable cadre of scholars who welcomed me and with whom I'm now pleased to work. Postdoctoral work with Jenny Reardon at the Science and Justice Research Center productively deepened my analyses of the intersections of race, gender, genomics, and their contemporary salience in science and technology studies (S&TS). At UC Santa Cruz, my colleagues at the Science and Justice Research Center, particularly the Race, Genomics, and Media Working Group, deserve special mention: Jenny Reardon, Herman Gray, Sandra Harvey, Maile Arvin, and Colleen

Stone. Our intensive collaboration, generative discussions, and critical mutuality greatly inform this book.

A 2016 visiting assistant professorship in the Department of Black Studies at UC Santa Barbara gave me the opportunity to facilitate undergraduate and graduate conversations that brought an S&TS perspective to questions of race, racism, and racialization. In particular, I cherish my discussions with Jeffrey Stewart, Ingrid Banks, and Howard Winant, and subsequent publication with Terence Keel and George Lipsitz. In grateful consequence, I offer a warm note of appreciation to those anonymous reviewers who pushed my thinking immeasurably toward black feminist and technoscientific scholarship in situating race and gender front and center in S&TS.

The National Center for Faculty Diversity and Development (NCFDD) provided excellent resources and guidance as I developed a self-directed writing platform embedded in creative accountability and a healthy work–life balance. A special shout goes out to Zakiya Luna, whose NCFDD-inspired Write-on-Site (WOS) writing group convened weekly in Berkeley until 2016, and which I facilitated until 2019. To my WOS colleagues Rosalynn Vega, Ugo Edu, Sandra Harvey, Victoria Massie, Ashwak Hauter, and Adeola Oni-Orisan—thank you all.

This book benefits in no small part from the remarkable editorial and copyediting contributions of Anitra Grisales and Andrew Murray. Andy conducted a master class in digital editing that left me better informed and quite excited about future writing projects. Thank you both for your considerable patience in the development of this book.

I extend my regards to Jason Weidemann and the reviewers at the University of Minnesota Press. Thank you, Jason, for your enthusiastic support of my project from day one. Your clear and steadfast guidance has made the publication process that much easier to negotiate.

Sweetness in the Blood reached its penultimate evolute due to a generous grant from a University of California Humanities Research Institute Junior Faculty Manuscript Development Workshop Award. The award funded the gathering of a panel of senior faculty who gave substantive feedback about the manuscript. I want to thank panel members Kelly Knight, Ingrid Banks, Carolyn Thomas, Herman Gray, and Damien Sojoyner for their participation and generative comments.

I am pleased and fortunate to have received generous funding throughout the course of researching and writing *Sweetness in the*

Blood: a University of California Chancellor's Fellowship; the Ford Foundation Dissertation Fellowship; the University of California President's Postdoctoral Fellowship; a University of California, Santa Cruz, Faculty Research Grant; and the University of California Humanities Research Institute Junior Faculty Manuscript Development Award.

I want to acknowledge with love my family near and far, without whom this book would not have taken its form or content. My deepest appreciation to my maternal grandparents, Victorin and Marion Doucet, who migrated from the cane fields of Bayou Têche to a better life in upstate New York. They lived through a time when young people my age were expected to labor in backbreaking toil, yet they nevertheless gave me space throughout my early life to read for days and write for weeks, so that I could think freely forever. *Merci*.

A Subversive Glossary

Admixture—A genetic parallel to hybridity and creolization that presumes the preexistence of biologically distinct groups and that views their combination as novel phenotypical forms.

Africanicity—Sub-Saharan DNA valued scientifically for its heterogeneity in a world that inversely devalues blackness as a biosocial threat to ethnoracial homogeneity.

Altruism—A form of sacrificial exchange obligated intersectionally according to race, gender, and socioeconomic status. It blurs the lines between agonist/donor, subject/citizen, and *ethnos/anthropos*.

Bioethics—A reworkable document of proscriptive research conduct one step behind the actual conditions of the laboratory and the field. As such, bioethical statements are historiographic, insufficiently ethnographic, rarely prescriptive or anticipatorily accurate, and conceptually pre-paradigmatic.

Black Church—A racialized but not monolithic social edifice of collective aspirations and appeals to justice, stratified by socioeconomic status, marked by imbalanced gendered participation, and characterized by clergy who lead from behind and not the front, of its congregations.

Cultural Competence—A desired subset of professional competence that struggles to keep pace with cultural change and highlights larger issues of locating expertise, trust, and expert authority.

Diaspora—Geographic dispersions of phenotypically similar groups marked spatially by diverse and often incongruent forms of cultural, environmental, and identitarian difference.

Gender—The biopolitical and bioeconomic engine driving the social and biological reproduction of society and the *Other*—a social, cultural, and political phenomenon largely absent from the archive; an independent variable that serves as a primary analytical site for examining the reproduction of kinship, race, and inequality.

Gift—Racial and gendered labor demanded without assured reciprocity as the conditional terms of citizenship and political inclusion, and which indexes social inequality; a necessary evil articulated as a moral duty in the name of progress.

Hope—An inculcated vision of future justice characterized by its violent absence in the present.

Internal Review Board (IRB)—Institutional review boards oversee the ethical conduct of research recruitment and protocols. As with post-Belmont and subsequent Common Rule policy implementations, IRBs tend to focus on the ethical relations between researchers and prospective individual participants. The necessary ethical commitments to communities and populations of scale remain relatively unaccompanied in IRB policies and requirements.

Matriarchy—An inherited right to resources and political influence through the female line; an ascripted label given to women of racialized lower socioeconomic classes; a false elevation in gendered social status that further *Others* those discursively embedded in these kinship groups in relational contrast to dominant patriarchal, ethnoracial, and socioeconomic structures.

Matrifocality—An intergenerational impoverishment dynamic based on a maternal-centered kinship structure characterized generally according to race and/or ethnicity by male exclusion from the wider socioeconomic field.

Prediabetes—An asymptomatic, liminal, and precursive state preceding a diabetes diagnosis. Diabetes risk scores and polygenetic diabetes risk scores imply a shift, respectively, from physiological risk to genetic risk. The genetic *pre-* in prediabetes has moved notions of risk further back in ancestral time.

Prediagnosis/Diagnosis—A collapsed temporal frame for determining the beginning of disease manifestation.

Race—A classificatory system of differentiated risks driven by political and economic forces that re-create new forms of biological value.

Recruitment—A perennial performance of making appeals to inclusive participation according to ethnicity, race, gender, socioeconomic status, and culture.

Refusal—Informed rejection of calls to enroll, submit, and participate in exchanges predicated upon ethnoracial and gendered categories of risk.

Reproduction—The biological regeneration of the gendered, socioeconomic, and political order that reconfigures the obligations of kinship, labor, and gift exchange.

Risk—A social, economic, and political balancing of the possible and the uncertain, leveraged by capital and embodied differently within and between social groups; a speculative engine driving research and markets.

Sacrificial Exchange—Socially and culturally embedded obligations to give without guarantee of reciprocity, a perennial precondition for racial and gendered inclusion.

Sugar—A historical commodity, metaphorical referent, embodied state, and nickname that emerged from the violent collision of globalizing capital, race, industrialization, and ethnocide.

Sweetness–Moments of possibility and delight hinted at and promised by sugar, betrayed punctually and metabolically by the absence of justice.

Thrifty Gene—An environmentally contingent genetic mechanism that drives diabetes risk independent of ethnicity or race.

Notes

INTRODUCTION

1. Gwendolyn Midlo Hall, *Africans in Colonial Louisiana: The Development of Afro-Creole Culture in the Eighteenth Century* (Baton Rouge: Louisiana State University Press, 1995).

2. Hall, *Africans in Colonial Louisiana.*

3. Jo Ann Carrigan, *The Saffron Scourge* (Lafayette: University of Louisiana at Lafayette Press, 2015).

4. The theoretical application of Hegelian dialectics to understanding former slave societies, by their descendants, begins with Du Bois and radiates through Fanon. Du Bois's "double consciousness" is, for Fanon, a "Manichaeism" dissonantly experienced subjectively and objectively. Marxian dialectics were not designed to analyze the colonial encounter; race, power, violence, and the ideology of difference trouble the relative social and racial homogeneity assumed within Marx's imaginaries. W. E. B. Du Bois, *The Souls of Black Folk* (Oxford: Oxford University Press, 2007 [1903]); Frantz Fanon, *The Wretched of the Earth* (New York: Grove, 1963); Frantz Fanon, *White Skin, Black Masks* (New York: Grove, 1968 [1952]).

5. Saidiya Hartman, *Lose Your Mother: A Journey Along the Atlantic Slave Route* (London: Macmillan, 2007).

6. Jessica Firger, "Sugar-Sweetened Beverages Are Now Cheaper than Bottled Water in Many Countries," *Newsweek,* May 4, 2017, https://www.newsweek.com/sugar-sweetened-beverages-soda-cheaper-obesity-cancer-diabetes-594827. Arguably, the sugar water of the plantation found its postmodern evolute in the creation of Gatorade, formulated for University of Florida Gator football players laboring under the hot Gainesville sun, at exactly the same time African Americans desegregated the team specifically and the Southeastern Conference (SEC) generally. Today, a plethora of sports and energy drinks, as well as pre- and post-training beverages, exist in a rapidly expanding twenty-first-century market of sweetened liquids advertised to carry us through arduous labor under the demands of capital.

7. See Michael Omi and Howard Winant, *Racial Formation in the United States: From the 1960s to the 1980s* (New York: Routledge and Kegan Paul, 2015).

8. Laura Nader, "Up the Anthropologist—Perspectives Gained from Studying Up," in *Reinventing Anthropology,* ed. Dell H. Hymes (New York: Pantheon, 1972), 284–311.

9. Natalia Aguilar Delgado and Luciano Barin Cruz, "Multi-event Ethnography: Doing Research in Pluralistic Settings," *Journal of Organizational Ethnography* 3, no. 1 (2014): 43–58; Bram Büscher, "Collaborative Event Ethnography: Between Structural Power and Empirical Nuance?," *Global Environmental Politics* 14, no. 3 (Aug 2014): 132–138.

10. New York State Department of Health, *Cirrhosis, Diabetes, and Kidney Indicators,* New York State Community Health Indicator Reports (CHIRS), 2016, https://webbi1.health.ny.gov/SASStoredProcess/guest?_program=%2FEBI%2FPHIG%2Fapps% 2Fchir_dashboard%2Fchir_dashboard&p=sh&stop=4. The Monroe County Coroner cannot keep pace with the number of fatal overdose victims requiring autopsy. The state flies in a second pathologist weekly to assist in reducing the backlog. See "Exclusive: Monroe County Testing Backlog Leaves Pain of Waiting for Families," WHEC, March 21, 2018, https://www.whec.com/news/me-office-backlog/4835452/.

11. Andrea Stuart, *Sugar in the Blood* (London: Portobello, 2012).

1. THE AT-RISK ETHNOGRAPHER OF SWEETNESS

1. Pseudonyms are used for most individual and institutional names throughout the text.

2. Ulrich Beck, "Living in the World Risk Society," *Economy and Society* 35, no. 3 (August 2006); Anthony Giddens, "Risk and Responsibility," *Modern Law Review* 62, no. 1 (January 1999); Nikolas Rose, *The Politics of Life Itself: Biomedicine, Power, and Subjectivity in the Twenty-First Century* (Princeton, N.J.: Princeton University Press, 2007); Mary Douglas and Aaron Wildavsky, *Risk and Culture: An Essay on the Selection of Technological and Environmental Dangers* (Berkeley: University of California Press, 1983); Frank Knight, *Risk, Uncertainty, and Profit* (Boston: Houghton Mifflin, 1921).

3. Annemarie Mol, *The Logic of Care* (New York: Routledge, 2009).

4. Sheila Jasanoff, ed., *States of Knowledge: The Co-Production of Science and the Social Order* (New York: Routledge Chapman & Hall, 2004).

5. Anthony Ryan Hatch, *Blood Sugar: Racial Pharmacology and Food Justice in Black America* (Minneapolis: University of Minnesota Press, 2016).

6. W. E. B. Du Bois, *Dusk of Dawn* (New York: Schocken, 1940); Catherine Waldby and Robert Mitchell, *Tissue Economies* (Durham, N.C.: Duke University Press, 2006); Nadia Abu El-Haj, "The Genetic Reinscription of Race," *Annual Review of Anthropology* 36 (2007).

7. Karl Marx, *Capital: A Critique of Political Economy* (London: Penguin, 2004); Karl Marx, *Grundrisse: Foundations of a Critique of Political Economy*

(London: Penguin, 1993); Georg Simmel, *The Philosophy of Money* (London: Taylor & Francis, 2011 [1900]); Karl Polanyi, *The Great Transformation* (Boston: Beacon Press, 1957); Jasanoff, *States of Knowledge.*

8. Douglas and Wildavsky, *Risk and Culture.*

9. Knight, *Risk, Uncertainty, and Profit.*

10. Beck, "World Risk Society."

11. Beck, "World Risk Society," 2–3; Beverly Woodward, "Challenges to Human Subject Protections in US Medical Research," *JAMA* 282, no. 2 (November 1999).

12. Du Bois, *Dusk of Dawn.*

13. Arleen Marcia Tuchman, "Diabetes and RACE A Historical Perspective," *American Journal of Public Health* 101, no. 1 (January 2011); Lundy Braun and Evelynn Hammonds, "The Dilemma of Classification," in *Genetics and the Unsettled Past*, ed. Keith Wailoo, Alondra Nelson, and Catherine Lee (New Brunswick, N.J.: Rutgers University Press, 2012); Lundy Braun, *Breathing Race Into the Machine* (Minneapolis: University of Minnesota Press, 2014).

14. Jeremy A. Greene, *Prescribing by Numbers: Drugs and the Definition of Disease* (Baltimore, Md.: Johns Hopkins University Press, 2007); Jonathan Xavier Inda, *Racial Prescriptions: Pharmaceuticals, Difference, and the Politics of Life* (New York: Routledge, 2014).

15. Troy Duster, "Medicalisation of Race," *The Lancet* 369, no. 9562 (February 24, 2007); Jonathan Kahn, *Race in a Bottle* (New York: Columbia University Press, 2012).

16. Steven Epstein, *Inclusion: The Politics of Difference in Medical Research* (Chicago: University of Chicago Press, 2008), 3–4.

17. Peter Lassman, Irving Velody, and Herminio Martins, *Max Weber's 'Science as a Vocation'* (London: Routledge, 2015); Duana Fullwiley, "Race and Genetics: Attempts to Define the Relationship," *BioSocieties* 2, no. 2 (June 2007): 236.

18. Michael J. Montoya, "Bioethnic Conscription: Genes, Race, and Mexicana/o Ethnicity in Diabetes Research," *Cultural Anthropology* 22, no. 1 (February 2007).

19. Epstein, *Inclusion*, 6–7.

20. Jonathan Marks, *Is Science Racist?* (Hoboken, N.J.: Wiley, 2017); Richard C. Lewontin, *Biology as Ideology: The Doctrine of DNA* (New York: Harper Collins, 1993).

21. Catherine Waldby, "Stem Cells, Tissue Cultures and the Production of Biovalue," *Health* 6, no. 3 (July 2002); Charis Thompson, *Making Parents: The Ontological Choreography of Reproductive Technologies* (Cambridge, Mass.: MIT Press, 2005); Charis Thompson, *Good Science: The Ethical Choreography of Stem Cell Research* (Cambridge, Mass.: MIT Press, 2013); Kaushik

Sunder Rajan, *Biocapital: The Constitution of Postgenomic Life* (Durham, N.C.: Duke University Press, 2006); Rose, *The Politics of Life Itself.*

22. Sunder Rajan, *Biocapital.*

23. Kean Birch and David Tyfield, "Theorizing the Bioeconomy: Biovalue, Biocapital, Bioeconomics or . . . What?," *Science, Technology, & Human Values* 38, no. 3 (May 2013): 301–2; cf. Melinda Cooper, *Life as Surplus: Biotechnology and Capitalism in the Neoliberal Era* (Seattle: University of Washington Press, 2008).

24. Cf. Arjun Appadurai, *The Social Life of Things: Commodities in Cultural Perspective* (Cambridge: Cambridge University Press, 1988); Susan Reynolds Whyte, Sjaak van der Geest, and Anita Hardon, *Social Lives of Medicines* (Cambridge: Cambridge University Press, 2002); Cori Hayden, *When Nature Goes Public: The Making and Unmaking of Bioprospecting in Mexico* (Princeton, N.J.: Princeton University Press, 2003).

25. Cf. Joseph Dumit, "A Pharmaceutical Grammar: Drugs for Life and Direct-to-Consumer Advertising in an Era of Surplus Health," unpublished paper, Department of Anthropology, University of California, Davis (2003).

26. Michael Morrison and Lucas Cornips, "Exploring the Role of Dedicated Online Biotechnology News Providers in the Innovation Economy," *Science, Technology, & Human Values* 37, no. 3 (May 2012); Beck, "World Risk Society."

27. Beck, "World Risk Society."

28. Whyte, van der Geest, and Hardon, *Social Lives of Medicines*; cf. Appadurai, *The Social Life of Things.*

29. A growing body of research examines sugar, creolization, and diabetes in the Indian Ocean. See Richard B. Allen, "Capital, Illegal Slaves, Indentured Labourers and the Creation of a Sugar Plantation Economy in Mauritius, 1810–60," *Journal of Imperial and Commonwealth History* (2008); François Vergès, "Indian-Oceanic Creolizations: Processes and Practices of Creolization on Réunion Island," in *Creolization: History, Ethnography, Theory,* ed. Charles Stewart (New York: Routledge, 2007). On the prevalence of diabetes in the wider South Asia, Indo-Pacific Region, see Arun Nanditha, Ronald C. W. Ma, Ambady Ramachandran, Chamukuttan Snehalatha, Juliana C. N. Chan, Kee Seng Chia, Jonathan E. Shaw, and Paul Z. Zimmet, "Diabetes in Asia and the Pacific: Implications for the Global Epidemic," *Diabetes Care* (2016).

30. Hall, *Africans in Colonial Louisiana*; Margaret M. Marshall, "The Origin and Development of Louisiana Creole French," in *French and Creole in Louisiana,* ed. Albert Valdman (New York: Springer, 1997).

31. Michel-Rolph Trouillot, "The Caribbean Region: An Open Frontier in Anthropological Theory," *Annual Review of Anthropology* 21 (1992); Brackette F. Williams, *Stains on My Name, War in My Veins: Guyana and the Politics of Cultural Struggle* (Durham, N.C.: Duke University Press, 1991).

32. Henry Hobhouse, *Seeds of Change: Five Plants That Changed the World* (London: Sidgwick & Jackson, 1985).

33. See Mintz's foreword to Jean Besson, *Martha Brae's Two Histories: European Expansions and Caribbean Culture-Building in Jamaica* (Chapel Hill: University of North Carolina Press, 2002), xvi. In Sharon Gmelch and George Gmelch, *The Parish Behind God's Back* (Long Grove, Ill.: Waveland, 2012), the "alien" social label is applied to U.S. African Americans, while the "exotic" is reserved for the Barbadians by both researchers and their students. Barbadian slavery induced a level of reflexivity and empathy previously not accorded to U.S. African Americans due to shared history, disparities in social status, and the unresolved nature of domestic race relations.

34. Melville Jean Herskovits, *The Myth of the Negro Past* (Boston: Beacon, 1990 [1941]).

35. Edouard Glissant, *Faulkner, Mississippi* (Chicago: University of Chicago Press, 1996), 29.

36. Paul Gilroy, *The Black Atlantic: Modernity and Double-Consciousness* (New York: Verso, 1993).

37. Paul Gilroy, *Against Race: Imagining Political Culture Beyond the Color Line* (Cambridge, Mass.: Harvard University Press, 2000).

38. James Clifford, *Routes: Travel and Translation in the Late Twentieth Century* (Cambridge, Mass.: Harvard University Press, 1997).

39. Eric Hobsbawm and Terence Ranger, *The Invention of Tradition* (Cambridge: Cambridge University Press, 2012); David Avrom Bell, *The Cult of the Nation in France: Inventing Nationalism, 1680–1800* (Cambridge, Mass.: Harvard University Press, 2001).

40. Clifford, *Routes*, 266–67. This is a syncretic process that Clifford, as read through Césaire, had earlier called "Caribbean." See: James Clifford, *The Predicament of Culture: Twentieth-Century Ethnography, Literature, and Art* (Cambridge, Mass.: Harvard University Press, 1988), 172–73.

41. Jacqueline Nassy Brown, *Dropping Anchor, Setting Sail: Geographies of Race in Black Liverpool* (Princeton, N.J.: Princeton University Press, 2009), 201.

42. Trouillot, "The Caribbean Region," 30.

43. Nassy Brown, *Dropping Anchor, Setting Sail*.

44. Viranjini Munasinghe, *Callaloo or Tossed Salad? East Indians and the Cultural Politics of Identity in Trinidad* (Ithaca, N.Y.: Cornell University Press, 2001), 136–39.

45. Aisha Khan, "Journey to the Center of the Earth: The Caribbean as Master Symbol," *Cultural Anthropology* 16, no. 3 (August 2001); Shalini Puri, *The Caribbean Postcolonial: Social Equality, Post/Nationalism, and Cultural Hybridity* (New York: Palgrave Macmillan, 2004).

46. Puri, *The Caribbean Postcolonial*.

47. Munasinghe, *Callaloo or Tossed Salad?*

48. Michael A. Gomez, *Exchanging Our Country Marks: The Transformation of African Identities in the Colonial and Antebellum South* (Chapel Hill: University of North Carolina Press, 1998).

49. Bill Maurer, "Ungrounding Knowledges Offshore: Caribbean Studies, Disciplinarity, and Critique," *Comparative American Studies* 2, no 3 (August 2004): 329. See also Bill Maurer, *Recharting the Caribbean: Land, Law, and Citizenship in the British Virgin Islands* (Ann Arbor: University of Michigan Press, 1997); Marilyn Strathern, "Future Kinship and the Study of Culture," *Futures* 27, no 4 (May 1995).

50. Maurer, "Ungrounding Knowledges Offshore," 329; Stephan Palmié, "Creolization and Its Discontents," *Annual Review of Anthropology* 35 (2006).

51. Montoya, "Bioethnic Conscription"; Yin C. Paradies, Michael J. Montoya, and Stephanie M. Fullerton, "Racialized Genetics and the Study of Complex Diseases: The Thrifty Genotype Revisited," *Perspectives in Biology and Medicine* 50, no. 2 (Spring 2007).

52. Charles L. Briggs and Daniel Hallin, "Biocommunicability: The Neoliberal Subject and Its Contradictions in News Coverage of Health Issues," *Social Text* 25, no. 493 (December 2007): 43–44.

53. Briggs and Hallin, "Biocommunicability," 46; Charles L. Briggs, "Communicability, Racial Discourse, and Disease," *Annual Review of Anthropology* 34 (2005): 270–71.

54. Elizabeth A. Povinelli, "Radical Worlds: The Anthropology of Incommensurability and Inconceivability," *Annual Review of Anthropology* 30 (2001): 325.

55. Bronislaw Malinowski, *Argonauts of the Western Pacific: An Account of Native Enterprise and Adventure in the Archipelagos of Melanesian New Guinea* (New York: Taylor & Francis, 2003 [1922]); Marcel Mauss, *The Gift: The Form and Reason for Exchange in Archaic Societies* (New York: Routledge, 1990 [1954]).

56. W. E. B. Du Bois, *The Gift of Black Folk: The Negroes in the Making of America* (Oxford: Oxford University Press, 1924); Marilyn Strathern, *The Gender of the Gift: Problems with Women and Problems with Society in Melanesia* (Berkeley: University of California Press, 1988).

57. Du Bois, *The Gift of Black Folk*; Mauss, *The Gift*.

58. Catherine Waldby, "Umbilical Cord Blood: From Social Gift to Venture Capital," *BioSocieties* 1, no. 1 (March 2006): 56–57.

59. Joan W. Scott, "Gender: A Useful Category of Historical Analysis," *American Historical Review* 91, no. 5 (December 1986).

60. Richard Hyland, "Gift and Danger," *Journal of Classical Sociology* 14, no. 1 (February 2014); Karla F. C. Holloway, *Legal Fictions: Constituting Race, Composing Literature* (Durham, N.C.: Duke University Press, 2014), x.

61. Hortense J. Spillers, "Mama's Baby, Papa's Maybe: An American Grammar Book," *Diacritics* 17, no. 2 (1987): 67.

62. Karla F. C. Holloway, *Private Bodies, Public Texts: Race, Gender, and a Cultural Bioethics* (Durham, N.C.: Duke University Press, 2011), 9.

63. Epstein, *Inclusion*, 6–7.

64. Alondra Nelson, "Bio Science: Genetic Genealogy Testing and the Pursuit of African Ancestry," *Social Studies of Science* 38, no. 5 (October 2008).

65. Cf. Deborah A. Bolnick, Duana Fullwiley, Troy Duster, Richard S. Cooper, Joan J. Fujimura, Jonathan Kahn, Jay S. Kaufman et al., "The Science and Business of Genetic Ancestry Testing," *Science* 318, no. 5849 (October 19, 2007); Nelson, "Bio Science."

66. Toni Morrison, *Beloved* (New York: Knopf, 1987).

67. Saidiya Hartman, *Lose Your Mother: A Journey Along the Atlantic Slave Route* (New York: Farrar, Straus, and Giroux, 2008), 16.

68. Saidiya Hartman, "Venus in Two Acts," *Small Axe: A Caribbean Journal of Criticism* 12, no. 2 (June 2008).

69. Spillers, "Mama's Baby, Papa's Maybe," 67.

70. Dorothy Roberts, *Killing the Black Body* (New York: Knopf Doubleday Publishing Group, 2014 [1997]); Spillers, "Mama's Baby, Papa's Maybe," 67.

71. Waldby, "Stem Cells."

72. W. E. B. Du Bois and Isabel Eaton, *The Philadelphia Negro: A Social Study* (Philadelphia: University of Pennsylvania Press, 1899); Benedict Anderson, *Imagined Communities: Reflections on the Origin and Spread of Nationalism* (New York: Verso, 2006 [1983]).

73. Montoya, "Bioethnic Conscription," 95.

74. *Race, the Floating Signifier*, directed by Sut Jhally, featuring Stewart Hall and Sut Jhally, Media Education Foundation, 1997, film.

75. Fullwiley, "Race and Genetics"; Duana Fullwiley, "The Molecularization of Race: Institutionalizing Human Difference in Pharmacogenetics Practice," *Science as Culture* 16, no. 1 (March 2007); Lundy Braun, Anne Fausto-Sterling, Duana Fullwiley, Evelynn M. Hammonds, Alondra Nelson, William Quivers, Susan M. Reverby, and Alexandra E. Shields, "Racial Categories in Medical Practice: How Useful Are They?," *PLOS Medicine* 4, no. 9 (September 2007).

76. Hatch, *Blood Sugar*.

77. Herskovits, *Myth of the Negro Past*.

2. SWEET BLOOD

1. Written in the third century BCE, the *Charaka Samhita*, one of the three main classical texts in Ayurvedic medicine, described the etiology, pathogenesis, symptomology, diagnosis, lines of treatment, and complications of

three main types and their myriad varieties of what we understand today as Type 2 diabetes. It should be noted that Charaka—known for his expository writing on internal medicine—classified diabetes, or *prāmeha,* as one of several "Obstinate Urinary Disorders." See Ram Karan Sharma and Vaidya Bhagwan Dash (translators), *Caraka Samhita. Text with English Translation & Critical Exposition Based on Cakrapāni Datta's Āyurveda Dīpikā, Volume 2* (Varanasi: Chowkhamba Sanskrit Series Office, 1985), 53–66.

2. I use the terms *obesogenic* and *diabetogenic* in terms of *genesis,* not *genetics.* Although much research has been and continues to occur in this area, I suggest no presumptive connection between obesity, T2D, and genetics.

3. The International Expert Committee (David M. Nathan, corresponding author), "International Expert Committee Report on the Role of the A1C Assay in the Diagnosis of Diabetes," *Diabetes Care* 32, no. 7 (July 2009).

4. Frank W. Booth and Darrell P. Neufer, "Exercise Controls Gene Expression: The Activity Level of Skeletal Muscle Modulates a Range of Genes That Produce Dramatic Molecular Changes—and Keep Us Healthy," *American Scientist* 93, no. 1 (January–February 2005); Anne D. Hafstad, Neoma Boardman, and Ellen Aasum, "How Exercise May Amend Metabolic Disturbances in Diabetic Cardiomyopathy," *Antioxidanta & Redox Signaling* 22, no. 17 (March 2015); Sheri R. Colberg, Ann L. Albright, Bryan J. Blissmer, Barry Braun, Lisa Chasan-Taber, Bo Fernhall, Judith G. Regensteiner et al., "Exercise and Type 2 Diabetes: The American College of Sports Medicine and the American Diabetes Association: Joint Position Statement," *Diabetes Care* 33, no. 12 (December 2010); Ronald J. Sigal, Glen P. Kenny, David H. Wasserman, Carmen Castaneda-Sceppa, and Russell D. White, "Physical Activity/Exercise and Type 2 Diabetes: A Consensus Statement from the American Diabetes Association," *Diabetes Care* 29, no. 6 (June 2006).

5. James V. Neel, "Diabetes Mellitus: A 'Thrifty' Genotype Rendered Detrimental by 'Progress'?," *American Journal of Human Genetics* 14, no. 4 (December 1962).

6. Neel, "Diabetes Mellitus," 360.

7. Margery Fee, "Racializing Narratives: Obesity, Diabetes and the 'Aboriginal' Thrifty Genotype," *Social Science & Medicine* 62, no. 12 (June 2006).

8. Neel, "Diabetes Mellitus," 359–60.

9. Thomas R. Dawber, Gilcin F. Meadors, and Felix E. Moore, "Epidemiological Approaches to Heart Disease: The Framingham Study," *American Journal of Public Health and the Nations Health,* 41, no. 3 (March 1951).

10. Dawber, Meadors, and Moore, "Epidemiological Approaches to Heart Disease," 281.

11. As chronicled by Landecker and later Skloot, Henrietta Lacks was an African American woman whose cervical cancer cells were collected by George Gey at Johns Hopkins University in 1952, which subsequently

revolutionized medical history and revitalized the discipline of cellular biology. Anonymized as "HeLa," the cell line was later commodified without the knowledge of the family at a time when informed consent was not yet a legal norm. See Hannah Landecker, "Immortality, In Vitro: A History of the HeLa Cell Line," in *Biotechnology and Culture: Bodies, Anxieties, Ethics,* ed. Paul Brodwin (Bloomington: Indiana University Press, 2000); Rebecca Skloot, *The Immortal Life of Henrietta Lacks* (New York: Broadway, 2011).

12. Edmund Leach, *Political Systems of Highland Burma: A Study of Kachin Social Structure* (Cambridge, Mass.: Harvard University Press, 1954).

13. Rohit Varma, Sylvia H. Paz, Stanley P. Azen, Ronald Klein, Denise Globe, Mina Torres, Chrisandra Shufelt, Susan Preston-Martin, and Los Angeles Latino Eye Study Group, "The Los Angeles Latino Eye Study: Design, Methods, and Baseline Data," *Ophthalmology* 111, no. 6 (June 2004): 1121.

14. Action to Control Cardiovascular Risk in Diabetes Study Group (ACCORD), Hertzel C. Gerstein, Michael E. Miller, Robert P. Byington, David C. Goff Jr, J. Thomas Bigger, John B. Buse et al., "Effects of Intensive Glucose Lowering in Type 2 Diabetes," *New England Journal of Medicine* 358, no. 24 (June 2008).

15. Varma et al., "The Los Angeles Latino Eye Study."

16. Kashif Mazhar, Rohit Varma, Farzana Choudhury, Roberta McKean-Cowdin, Corina J. Shtir, Stanley P. Azen, and the Los Angeles Latino Eye Study Group, "Severity of Diabetic Retinopathy and Health-Related Quality of Life: The Los Angeles Latino Eye Study," *Ophthalmology* 118, no. 4 (April 2011).

17. U.S. Indian Bureau, "River People, Pima Indians of Arizona," F. C. Clark, director (1948), https://www.youtube.com/watch?v=RZfA0ucMCGA; Office of Indian Affairs, "Supai Indian," David Smart, producer, Periscope Films, (1945), https://www.youtube.com/watch?v=N2ftZzGUtxA; see also "The Navajo Indian," revised version of 1945 film (Coronet Instructional Media, 1975), http://archive.org/details/thenavajoindian.

18. In the interest of ethical transparency, note the absent attribution of full names in the production of these films.

19. Leslie J. Baier and Robert L. Hanson, "Genetic Studies of the Etiology of Type 2 Diabetes in Pima Indians: Hunting for Pieces to a Complicated Puzzle," *Diabetes* 53, no. 5 (May 2004); B. L. Hanna, A. A. Dahlberg, and H. H. Strandskov, "A Preliminary Study of the Population History of the Pima Indians," *American Journal of Human Genetics* 5, no. 4 (December 1953).

20. Mette Korre Andersen, Casper-Emil Tingskov Pedersen, Ida Moltke, Torben Hansen, Anders Albrechtsen, and Niels Grarup, "Genetics of Type 2 Diabetes: The Power of Isolated Populations," *Current Diabetes Reports* 16, no. 7 (2016): 65.

21. Rex Dalton, "When Two Tribes Go to War," *Nature* (news), July 8, 2004, 500, https://www.nature.com/articles/430500a.

22. David Usborne, "Blood Feud in the Grand Canyon," *The Independent*, April 23, 2010, http://www.independent.co.uk/news/world/americas/blood-feud-in-the-grand-canyon-1951972.html. The principle researcher, an evolutionary biologist, no longer lists her previous research among the Havasupai.

23. Usborne, "Blood Feud in the Grand Canyon."

24. Herman Gray, "Subject(Ed) to Recognition," *American Quarterly* 65, no. 4 (December 2013).

25. Vandana Shiva, *Biopiracy: The Plunder of Nature and Knowledge* (Berkeley, Calif.: North Atlantic, 2016); Jenny Reardon and Kim TallBear, "'Your DNA Is Our History': Genomics, Anthropology, and the Construction of Whiteness as Property," *Current Anthropology* 53, no. S5 (April 2011).

26. See Alondra Nelson, "Bio Science: Genetic Genealogy Testing and the Pursuit of African Ancestry," *Social Studies of Science* 38, no. 5 (October 1, 2008): 759–83. Nelson demonstrated that even when ethnographic data showed subjective confusion about race, both in terms of personal and social meaning, genetics researchers bracketed out such understandings in the face of research protocols based on objectively constructed racial categories.

27. Arleen Marcia Tuchman, "Diabetes and Race: A Historical Perspective," *American Journal of Public Health* 101, no. 1 (January 1, 2011): 24–33.

28. Tuchman, "Diabetes and Race"; Michael Montoya, *Making the Mexican Diabetic: Race, Science, and the Genetics of Inequality* (Berkeley: University of California Press, 2011).

29. R. Havelock Charles, Rai Koilas Chunder Bose, C. L. Bose, Satyasaran Chakravarti, Rai Devendranath Roy, and F. M. Sandwith, "Discussion on Diabetes in the Tropics," *British Medical Journal* 2, no. 2442 (October 19, 1907): 1051–64. Professor Hans Ziemann argued that a diet based on plantains and cassava, but not rice, resulted in no clinical evidence of diabetes in the Cameroons (1061). Other discussants, particularly from India and Ceylon (Sri Lanka), found a high prevalence of diabetes among vegetarians, Brahmins, merchants, and those others eating a mostly rice-based, high-carbohydrate, low-protein diet. Exacerbated by a sedentary lifestyle, these dietary factors increased diabetes risk, which led some South Asian discussants to suggest culturally appropriate and more nutritious substitutes to decrease rice consumption.

30. Hugh Payne Greeley, "Habit versus Instinct in Eating," *Boston Medical and Surgical Journal* 179, no. 25 (December 1918).

31. A. G. Love and C. B. Davenport, "A Comparison of White and Colored Troops in Respect to Incidence of Disease," *Proceedings of the National Academy of Sciences of the United States of America* 5, no. 3 (March 1919): 60.

32. W. E. B. Du Bois, *Dusk of Dawn: An Essay Toward an Autobiography of a Race Concept* (New York: Schocken, 1940).

33. Mary C. Waters, *Black Identities* (Cambridge, Mass.: Harvard University Press, 1999).

34. See Kimberlé Crenshaw, "Demarginalizing the Intersection of Race and Sex: A Black Feminist Critique of Antidiscrimination Doctrine, Feminist Theory and Antiracist Politics," *University of Chicago Legal Forum* 1989 (1989).

35. The terms *metabolic syndrome* and *cardiometabolic syndrome* are used almost interchangeably; therefore, the cardiometabolic pathology is not seen as sequelae to the metabolic syndrome. Unless otherwise specified, I will employ the more descriptive term *cardiometabolic syndrome*.

36. See Du Bois, *Dusk of Dawn*; Franz Boas, *Race and Democratic Society* (New York: J. J. Augustin, 1945).

37. Yin C. Paradies, Michael J. Montoya, and Stephanie M. Fullerton, "Racialized Genetics and the Study of Complex Diseases: The Thrifty Genotype Revisited," *Perspectives in Biology and Medicine* 50, no. 2 (2007): 203–27; Fee, "Racializing Narratives."

38. Dawber, Meadors, and Moore, "Epidemiological Approaches to Heart Disease," 279.

39. For a more global confirmation, see Paul Z. Zimmet, "Diabetes and Its Drivers: The Largest Epidemic in Human History?" *Clinical Diabetes and Endocrinology* 3, no. 1 (January 18, 2017): 1.

40. Centers for Disease Control and Prevention, *National Diabetes Statistics Report* (Washington, D.C.: National Center for Chronic Disease Prevention and Health Promotion, Division of Diabetes Translation, July 18, 2017), https://www.cdc.gov/diabetes/pdfs/data/statistics/national-diabetes-statistics-report.pdf.

41. Vanita R. Aroda and Robert Ratner, "Approach to the Patient with Prediabetes," *Journal of Clinical Endocrinology & Metabolism* 93, no. 9 (September 2008).

42. Stephanie M. Benjamin, Rodolfo Valdez, Linda S. Geiss, Deborah B. Rolka, and K. M. Venkat Narayan, "Estimated Number of Adults with Prediabetes in the U.S. in 2000: Opportunities for Prevention," *Diabetes Care* 26, no. 3 (March 2003); Aaron Vinik, "Advancing Therapy in Type 2 Diabetes Mellitus with Early, Comprehensive Progression from Oral Agents to Insulin Therapy," *Clinical Therapeutics* 29, no. 6 Pt 1 (June 2007).

43. Jeremy A. Greene, *Prescribing by Numbers: Drugs and the Definition of Disease* (Baltimore, Md.: Johns Hopkins University Press, 2007).

44. "Reports from Meetings," *Acta Diabetologia Latina* 12, no. 3 (May 1975); B. Schulz, S. Knospe, D. Michaelis, K. Titze, and W. Hildmann, "Relationship between Carbohydrate Tolerance, Insulin Secretion, and Insulin

Sensitivity of Isolated Fat Cells from Obese Protodiabetics," *Acta Diabetologia Latina* 15, no. 3 (May 1978).

45. "Reports from Meetings," 248.

46. E. F. Pfeiffer and H. Laube, "Obesity and Diabetes Mellitus," *Advances in Metabolic Disorders* 7 (January 1974).

47. E. F. Pfeiffer, "Obesity, Hyperinsulinism and Diabetes Mellitus: Facts and Hypotheses," *Proceedings of the Royal Society of Medicine* 62 (April 1969).

48. Lorena Madrigal, *The Human Biology of Afro-Caribbean Populations* (Cambridge: University of Cambridge Press, 2006); Ian Whitmarsh, "Biomedical Ambivalence: Asthma Diagnosis, the Pharmaceutical, and Other Contradictions in Barbados," *American Ethnologist* 35, no. 1 (February 2008).

49. Paradies, Montoya, and Fullerton, "Racialized Genetics"; Michael J. Montoya, "Bioethnic Conscription: Genes, Race, and Mexicana/o Ethnicity in Diabetes Research." *Cultural Anthropology* 22, no. 1 (February 1, 2007): 94–128; For a fuller treatment, see Montoya, *Making the Mexican Diabetic.*

50. Whitmarsh, "Biomedical Ambivalence"; Michel S. Laguerre, *Afro-Caribbean Folk Medicine* (Granby, Mass.: Bergin & Garvey, 1987); cf. Kaushik Sunder Rajan, *Biocapital: The Constitution of Postgenomic Life* (Durham, N.C.: Duke University Press, 2006); cf. Adriana Petryna and Arthur Kleinman, "The Pharmaceutical Nexus," in *Global Pharmaceuticals: Ethics, Markets, Practices,* ed. Adriana Petryna, Andrew Lakoff, and Arthur Kleinman (Durham, N.C.: Duke University Press, 2006).

51. Ian Whitmarsh, *Biomedical Ambiguity: Race, Asthma, and the Contested Meaning of Genetic Research in the Caribbean* (Ithaca, N.Y.: Cornell University Press, 2008).

52. Sarah Franklin, "Ethical Biocapital: New Strategies of Cell Culture," in *Remaking Life and Death: Toward an Anthropology of the Biosciences,* ed. Sarah Franklin and Margaret Lock (Santa Fe, N.Mex.: School of American Research Press, 2003).

53. Franklin, "Ethical Biocapital," 61.

54. See also David Edgerton, "Creole Technologies and Global Histories: Rethinking How Things Travel in Space and Time," *History of Science and Technology* 1, no. 1 (2007): 75–112.

55. Lucy Suchman, "Feminist STS and the Sciences of the Artificial," in *Handbook of Science and Technology Studies,* ed. Edward J. Hackett, Olga Amsterdamska, Michael Lynch, and Judy Wajcman (Cambridge, Mass.: MIT Press, 2008).

56. Whitmarsh, "Biomedical Ambivalence"; Whitmarsh, *Biomedical Ambiguity,* 50; Steven Epstein, *Inclusion: The Politics of Difference in Medical Research* (Chicago: University of Chicago Press, 2008).

57. Cf. Jeremy A. Greene, "Pharmaceutical Marketing Research and the

Prescribing Physician," *Annals of Internal Medicine* 146, no. 10 (May 2007); cf. Greene, *Prescribing by Numbers.*

58. Biomarkers Definitions Working Group 2001, "Biomarkers and Surrogate Endpoints: Preferred Definitions and Conceptual Framework," *Clinical Pharmacology and Therapeutics* 69, no. 3 (March 2001).

59. American Diabetes Association, "Diagnosis and Classification of Diabetes Mellitus," *Diabetes Care* 33, supplement 1 (January 2010).

60. The Troglitazone group was disbanded after a research subject suffered liver failure and consequently died post–transplant surgery.

61. American Diabetes Association, "The Diabetes Prevention Program. Design and Methods for a Clinical Trial in the Prevention of Type 2 Diabetes," *Diabetes Care* 22, no. 4 (April 1999): 623–25.

62. American Diabetes Association, "Diabetes Prevention Program," 623.

63. National Academies of Sciences, Engineering, and Medicine, *The Challenge of Treating Obesity and Overweight: Proceedings of a Workshop* (Washington, D.C.: National Academies of Sciences, Engineering, and Medicine, 2017).

64. John P. Bantle, Judith Wylie-Rosett, Ann L. Albright, Caroline M. Apovian, Nathaniel G. Clark, Marion J. Franz, Byron J. Hoogwerf et al., "Nutrition Recommendations and Interventions for Diabetes-2006: A Position Statement of the American Diabetes Association," *Diabetes Care* 29, no. 9 (September 2006); American Diabetes Association, John P. Bantle, Judith Wylie-Rosett, Ann L. Albright, Caroline M. Apovian, Nathaniel G. Clark, Marion J. Franz et al., "Nutrition Recommendations and Interventions for Diabetes: A Position Statement of the American Diabetes Association," *Diabetes Care* 31, supplement 1 (January 2008).

65. Mova Leung, Debbie Kwan, and Michael F. Evans, "Lifestyle Intervention or Treatment with Metformin. Which Delays Onset of Type 2 Diabetes?," *Canadian Family Physician* 50 (2004): 369.

66. Chris Slentz, Lori A. Bateman, Leslie H. Willis, Esther O. Granville, Lucy W. Piner, Gregory P. Samsa, Tracy L. Setji et al., "Effects of Exercise Training Alone vs. a Combined Exercise and Nutritional Lifestyle Intervention on Glucose Homeostasis in Prediabetic Individuals: A Randomised Controlled Trial," *Diabetologia* 59, no. 10 (October 2016); Natalie Eichner, Julian M. Gaitán, Nicole M. Gilbertson, Mahnoor Khurshid, Arthur Weltman, and Steven K. Malin, "Postprandial Augmentation Index Is Reduced in Adults with Prediabetes Following Continuous and Interval Exercise Training," *Experimental Physiology* 104, no. 2 (2019).

67. Institute of Medicine of the National Academies, *Adequacy of Evidence for Physical Activity Guidelines Development: Workshop Summary* (Washington, D.C.: National Academies Press, 2007).

68. Caroline Trapp, Neal Barnard, and Heather Katcher, "A Plant-Based Diet for Type 2 Diabetes: Scientific Support and Practical Strategies," *Diabetes Educator* 36, no. 1 (January–February 2010); Neal D. Barnard, Joshua Cohen, David J. A. Jenkins, Gabrielle Turner-McGrievy, Lise Gloede, Brent Jaster, Kim Seidl, Amber A. Green, and Stanley Talpers, "A Low-Fat Vegan Diet Improves Glycemic Control and Cardiovascular Risk Factors in a Randomized Clinical Trial in Individuals with Type 2 Diabetes," *Diabetes Care* 29, no. 8 (August 2006).

69. Muriel Lily and Marshall Godwin, "Treating Prediabetes with Metformin: Systematic Review and Meta-analysis," *Canadian Family Physician* 55, no. 4 (April 2009).

70. Peter Bo Poulsen, *Health Technology Assessment and Diffusion of Health Technology,* (Odense: Syddansk Universitetsforlag, 1999).

71. National Academies of Sciences, Engineering, and Medicine, *The Challenge of Treating Obesity;* J. B. Dixon, P. Zimmet, K. G. Alberti, F. Rubino, and International Diabetes Federation Taskforce on Epidemiology and Prevention, "Bariatric Surgery: An IDF Statement for Obese Type 2 Diabetes," *Diabetic Medicine* 28, no. 6 (April 2011).

72. J. Picot, J. Jones, J. L. Colquitt, E. Gospodarevskaya, E. Loveman, L. Baxter, and A. J. Clegg, "The Clinical Effectiveness and Cost-Effectiveness of Bariatric (Weight Loss) Surgery for Obesity: A Systematic Review and Economic Evaluation," *Health Technology Assessment* 13, no. 41 (September 2009).

73. Jay S. Skyler, Richard Bergenstal, Robert O. Bonow, John Buse, Prakash Deedwania, Edwin A. M. Gale, Barbara V. Howard et al., "Intensive Glycemic Control and the Prevention of Cardiovascular Events: Implications of the ACCORD, ADVANCE, and VA Diabetes Trials: A Position Statement of the American Diabetes Association and a Scientific Statement of the American College of Cardiology Foundation and the American Heart Association," *Circulation* 119, no. 2 (January 2009).

74. See Greene, *Prescribing by Numbers* for a larger treatment on the development of Orinase.

75. Lily and Godwin, "Treating Prediabetes with Metformin," 352.

76. Lily and Godwin, "Treating Prediabetes with Metformin," 352.

77. Lily and Godwin, "Treating Prediabetes with Metformin," 355.

78. Amir Qaseem, Timothy J. Wilt, Devan Kansagara, Carrie Horwitch, Michael J. Barry, Mary Ann Forciea, and Clinical Guidelines Committee of the American College of Physicians, "Hemoglobin A1c Targets for Glycemic Control with Pharmacologic Therapy for Nonpregnant Adults with Type 2 Diabetes Mellitus: A Guidance Statement Update from the American College of Physicians," *Annals of Internal Medicine* 168, no. 8 (April 2018).

79. American Diabetes Association, "Glycemic Targets: Standards of Medical Care in Diabetes—2018," *Diabetes Care* 41, supplement 1 (January 2018).

80. American Diabetes Association, "Glycemic Targets."

81. Joseph Dumit, "Prescription Maximization and the Accumulation of Surplus Health in the Pharmaceutical Industry: The_BioMarx_Experiment," in *Lively Capital: Biotechnology, Ethics, and Governance in Global Markets,* ed. Kaushik Sunder Rajan (Durham, N.C.: Duke University Press, 2012); Joseph Dumit, *Drugs for Life: How Pharmaceutical Companies Define Our Health* (Durham, N.C.: Duke University Press, 2012).

82. Several publications in the first decade of the century noted this trend. See Troy Duster, "Medicalisation of Race," *The Lancet* 369, no. 9562 (February 24, 2007); Paradies, Montoya, and Fullerton, "Racialized Genetics."

3. ALGORITHMS OF RISK AND RACE

1. Bernadette Tansey, "Emeryville Firm Devises Diabetes Risk Test," *SFGate,* May 27, 2008, https://www.sfgate.com/business/article/Emeryville-firm-devises-diabetes-risk-test-3211853.php.

2. See Joseph Dumit, *Picturing Personhood: Brain Scans and Biomedical Identity* (Princeton, N.J.: Princeton University Press, 2004).

3. Evelynn M. Hammonds, "New Technologies of Race" in *Processed Lives: Gender and Technology in Everyday Life,* ed. Melodie Calvert and Jennifer Terry (New York: Routledge, 1997).

4. Jaana Lindström and Jaakko Tuomilehto, "The Diabetes Risk Score: A Practical Tool to Predict Type 2 Diabetes Risk," *Diabetes Care* 26, no. 3 (March 2003); E. 't Riet Van, M. Alssema, G. Nijpels, and J. M. Dekker, "Estimating the Individual Risk of Diabetes: Not on the Grounds of Overweight Only," *Nederlands tijdschrift voor geneeskunde* 152, no. 44 (November 2008).

5. V. Mohan, R. Deepa, M. Deepa, S. Somannavar, and M. Datta, "A Simplified Indian Diabetes Risk Score for Screening for Undiagnosed Diabetic Subjects," *Journal of the Association of Physicians of India* 53 (September 2005).

6. Robyn J. Tapp, Paul Z. Zimmet, C. Alex Harper, Daniel J. McCarty, Pierrot Chitson, Andrew M. Tonkin, Stefan Söderberg et al., "Six Year Incidence and Progression of Diabetic Retinopathy: Results from the Mauritius Diabetes Complication Study," *Diabetes Research and Clinical Practice* 73, no. 3 (September 2006).

7. Margery Fee, "Racializing Narratives: Obesity, Diabetes and the 'Aboriginal' Thrifty Genotype," *Social Science & Medicine* 62, no. 12 (June 1, 2006): 2988–97.

8. Primary and Mental Health Care Division, Australian Government

Department of Health, "Background to the Australian Type 2 Diabetes Risk Assessment Tool (AUSDRISK)," 2013, https://www.health.gov.au/internet/main/publishing.nsf/Content/chronic-diab-prev-aus-exp.

9. Diabetes UK, "Welcome to the Diabetes Risk Score," 2011, http://www.diabetes.org.uk/Riskscore/ (currently accessible as it appeared June 20, 2012, via https://web.archive.org/web/20120620180240/http://riskscore.diabetes.org.uk/). The website has since been updated, and the page describing risk factors now features references to African and Afro-Caribbean groups. See Diabetes UK, "Diabetes Risk Factors," https://www.diabetes.org.uk/preventing-type-2-diabetes/diabetes-risk-factors.

10. The University of Arizona and Arizona State University's BIO5 Institute is developing an alternative diabetes risk prediction model. See Johnny Cruz, "BIO5 and Biodesign Institutes Seek Early Detection of Type 2 Diabetes," *UANews*, October 3, 2007, https://uanews.arizona.edu/story/bio5-and-biodesign-institutes-seek-early-detection-of-type-2-diabetes.

11. Mickey Urdea, Janice Kolberg, Judith Wilber, Robert Gerwien, Edward Moler, Michael Rowe, Paul Jorgensen et al., "Validation of a Multimarker Model for Assessing Risk of Type 2 Diabetes from a Five-Year Prospective Study of 6784 Danish People (Inter99)," *Journal of Diabetes Science and Technology* 3, no. 4 (July 2009).

12. Charis Thompson, *Good Science: The Ethical Choreography of Stem Cell Research* (Cambridge, Mass.: MIT Press, 2013).

13. This interview occurred in 2009 before the passage of the Affordable Care Act (ACA) on March 23, 2010. The current government insurance co-pay plans offer four tiers of coverage, ranging from 10 to 40 percent out-of-pocket patient expenses. Therefore, the ACA changed some but not all the economic dynamics of Type 2 diabetes.

14. Centers for Disease Control and Prevention, "More than 29 Million Americans Have Diabetes; 1 in 4 Doesn't Know," 2014, https://www.cdc.gov/media/releases/2014/p0610-diabetes-report.html.

15. John Lie, *Multiethnic Japan* (Cambridge, Mass.: Harvard University Press, 2009); Richard Jenkins, *Being Danish: Paradoxes of Identity in Everyday Life* (Copenhagen: Museum Tusculanum Press, 2011).

16. Steven Epstein, *Inclusion: The Politics of Difference in Medical Research* (Chicago: University of Chicago Press, 2008); Jenny Reardon, *Race to the Finish: Identity and Governance in an Age of Genomics* (Princeton, N.J.: Princeton University Press, 2009).

17. Troy Duster, "Medicalisation of Race." *The Lancet* 369, no. 9562 (February 24, 2007): 702–4; Jonathan Kahn, *Race in a Bottle: The Story of BiDil and Racialized Medicine in a Post-Genomic Age* (New York: Columbia University Press, 2013).

18. Steven Epstein, "The Rise of 'Recruitmentology': Clinical Research, Racial Knowledge, and the Politics of Inclusion and Difference," *Social Studies of Science* 38, no. 5 (October 2008).

19. Arleen Marcia Tuchman, "Diabetes and Race: A Historical Perspective." *American Journal of Public Health* 101, no. 1 (January 1, 2011): 24–33; Lundy Braun, Anne Fausto-Sterling, Duana Fullwiley, Evelynn M. Hammonds, Alondra Nelson, William Quivers, Susan M. Reverby, and Alexandra E. Shields, "Racial Categories in Medical Practice: How Useful Are They?" *PLOS Medicine* 4, no. 9 (September 25, 2007): e271; Lundy Braun, *Breathing Race into the Machine: The Surprising Career of the Spirometer from Plantation to Genetics* (Minneapolis: University of Minnesota Press, 2014).

20. Jeremy A. Greene, *Prescribing by Numbers: Drugs and the Definition of Disease* (Baltimore, Md.: Johns Hopkins University Press, 2007).

21. Urdea et al., "Validation of a Multimarker Model."

22. While Walgreens is the largest retail drug store chain with the highest revenues, CVS Caremark administers pharmaceutical programs and services to over two thousand companies and government agencies representing nearly fifty-three million U.S. citizens. In 2008, Walgreens balked at honoring CVS Caremark clients' prescriptions less than four months before the Step Out! Against Diabetes Walk. The issue was settled, but after much mutual recrimination.

23. In subsequent years, the Oakland Step Out! Against Diabetes Walk has been held on Saturdays and relocated from Jack London Square to Lake Merritt. The circumference of Lake Merritt is three miles.

24. See Declan Butler, "Translational Research: Crossing the Valley of Death," *Nature* 453, no. 7197 (June 2008).

25. The passing of the Bayh-Dole Act in 1980 permitted universities and nonprofit organizations to obtain intellectual property (IP) rights from all federally funded research. This is the thirty-year period framing this conversation.

26. In many respects Genentech institutionalized the relationship between biotechnology and venture capital. See William A. Sahlman, "The Structure and Governance of Venture Capital Organizations," *Journal of Financial Economics* 27, no. 2 (October 1990); also, Walter W. Powell, Kenneth W. Koput, James I. Bowie, and Laurel Smith-Doerr, "Spatial Clustering of Science and Capital: Accounting for Biotech Firm-Venture Capital Relationships," *Regional Studies* 36, no. 3 (May 2002). The authors situate biotechnology's lifeblood in the dual streams of basic science and venture capital, which Genentech epitomizes and from which it emerged.

27. Genentech Hall, completed in 2002, was the first building of UC San Francisco's research-focused Mission Bay Campus. It was named following a

nine-year patent dispute between UCSF and Genentech over the drug Pro-tropin®. Part of the $200 million settlement in UCSF's favor included $50 million for the new building's construction. Genentech, however, received naming rights, and the company opted to name the new building after itself. See Katherine Weatherford Darling et al., "Just Biomedicine on Third Street? Health & Wealth Inequities in San Francisco's Biotech Hub," in *Counterpoints: A San Francisco Bay Area Atlas of Displacement & Resistance,* ed. Anti-Eviction Mapping Project (Oakland, Calif.: PM Press, forthcoming 2020).

28. See David Bornstein, "Helping New Drugs Out of Research's 'Valley of Death,'" *New York Times Opinionator,* May 2, 2011, http://opinionator .blogs.nytimes.com/2011/05/02/helping-new-drugs-out-of-academias -valley-of-death.

29. In *Seeing Like a State,* David C. Scott argued that state engineering of the social is predicated upon (1) the administrative ordering of nature; (2) the mastering of nature, both biological and human, through epistemic confidence in the telos of scientific and technological progress to address and satisfy human needs; (3) a state ready and able to deploy power authorita-tively and without reservation in actualizing the preceding objectives; and the last, vital element, (4) successful state-run social engineering of a submis-sive civil society unable to resist such plans. See David C. Scott, *Seeing Like a State: How Certain Schemes to Improve the Human Condition Have Failed* (New Haven, Conn.: Yale University Press, 1998), 4–5.

30. Joseph Dumit argues that pharmaceutical company marketing designs have shifted from a model based on "inherent health" to "inherent illness." "Health" and "normalcy" are now seen as pharmaceutically enabled, a life-long challenge, and predictable source of future market profitability. See Jo-seph Dumit, *Drugs for Life: How Pharmaceutical Companies Define Our Health* (Durham, N.C.: Duke University Press, 2012).

31. Susan Ward, "Demographic Factors in the Chinese Health-Care Market," *Nature Reviews Drug Discovery* 7 (May 2008): 383; Ronald Ching Wan Ma, Xu Lin, and Weiping Jia, "Causes of Type 2 Diabetes in China," *The Lancet Diabetes & Endocrinology* 2, no. 12 (December 2014); Cheng Hu and Weiping Jia, "Diabetes in China: Epidemiology and Genetic Risk Factors and Their Clinical Utility in Personalized Medication," *Diabetes* 67, no. 1 (Janu-ary 2018).

32. Sumedh S. Hoskote and Shashank R. Joshi, "Are Indians Destined to Be Diabetic?," *Journal of the Association of Physicians of India* 56 (April 2008).

33. Ward, "Demographic Factors in the Chinese Health-Care Market"; Hoskote and Joshi, "Are Indians Destined to Be Diabetic?"

34. Cf. Shruti Kapila, "Race Matters: Orientalism and Religion, India and Beyond c. 1770–1880," *Modern Asian Studies* 41, no. 3 (May 2007).

35. Deepa S. Reddy, "The Ethnicity of Caste," *Anthropological Quarterly* 78, no. 3 (August 2005).

36. Indian populations form part of a wider "South Asian" research category that has gained currency over the last several decades. In the case of Trinidad, Guyana, and to a lesser extent Suriname, immigrant Indian populations from various parts of north, east, and south India have collapsed into a generic "Indian" biopolitical category.

37. Wolfgang Rathmann, Bernd Kowall, and Matthias B. Schulze, "Development of a Type 2 Diabetes Risk Model from a Panel of Serum Biomarkers from the Inter99 Cohort: Response to Kolberg et al.," *Diabetes Care* 33, no. 2 (February 2010): e28.

38. Rathmann, Kowall, and Schulze, "Development of a Type 2 Diabetes Risk Model: Response to Kolberg et al."

39. Robert W. Gerwien, Michael W. Rowe, Edward Moler, Mickey S. Urdea, Michael P. McKenna, and Janice A. Kolberg, "Development of a Type 2 Diabetes Risk Model From a Panel of Serum Biomarkers From the Inter99 Cohort: Response to Rathmann, Kowall, and Schulze," *Diabetes Care* 33, no. 2 (February 2010): e29.

40. Gerwien et al., "Development of a Type 2 Diabetes Risk Model: Response to Rathmann, Kowall, and Schulze."

41. Steven E. F. Brown, "Air Force to Use Tethys Bioscience Blood Test in Diabetes Study," *San Francisco Business Times,* March 24, 2011, https://www.bizjournals.com/sanfrancisco/news/2011/03/24/air-force-to-use-tethys-bioscience.html.

42. Kean Birch and David Tyfield, "Theorizing the Bioeconomy: Biovalue, Biocapital, Bioeconomics or . . . What?" *Science, Technology, & Human Values* 38, no. 3 (May 1, 2013): 299–327; cf. Melinda E. Cooper and Catherine Waldby, *Life as Surplus: Biotechnology and Capitalism in the Neoliberal Era* (Seattle: University of Washington Press, 2011); and Melinda E. Cooper and Catherine Waldby, *Clinical Labor: Tissue Donors and Research Subjects in the Global Bioeconomy* (Durham, N.C.: Duke University Press, 2014).

43. Jonathan Norris, "Continued Rebound: Trends in Life Sciences Mergers & Acquisitions," *Silicon Valley Bank* (July 2012).

44. Michael W. Rowe, Richard N. Bergman, Lynne E. Wagenknecht, and Janice A. Kolberg, "Performance of a Multi-marker Diabetes Risk Score in the Insulin Resistance Atherosclerosis Study (IRAS), a Multi-ethnic US Cohort," *Diabetes/Metabolism Research and Reviews* 28, no. 6 (September 2012).

45. Bruce Booth, "Unhealthy Prognosis for Venture-Backed Diagnostics," *Life Sci VC* (April 27, 2013), https://lifescivc.com/2013/04/unhealthy-prognosis-for-venture-backed-diagnostics/.

46. Denial of Medicare reimbursement for PreDx™ DRS testing in 2013

eliminated a vital revenue stream for the company. See Cromwell Schubarth, "$100M Startup Tethys BioScience Seen Shutting Down," *Silicon Valley Business Journal,* November 4, 2013, https://www.bizjournals.com/sanjose/news/2013/11/04/100m-startup-tethys-bioscience-seen.html. In a last-ditch effort to recoup losses, former customers/patients found themselves receiving invoices in 2014, after the company ceased operations, for tests conducted upwards of four years earlier. They maintain that physicians assured them that insurance would cover the test. For a larger discussion, see Cafepharma (forum), "Tethys Bioscience," *Cafepharma Message Boards* ("Tell Me About Your Company"), 2010, http://www.cafepharma.com/boards/threads/tethys-bioscience.429881/.

47. Kaushik Sunder Rajan, *Biocapital: The Constitution of Postgenomic Life* (Durham, N.C.: Duke University Press, 2006), 6.

48. Braun, *Breathing Race into the Machine*; Annemarie Jutel and Sarah Nettleton, "Towards a Sociology of Diagnosis: Reflections and Opportunities," *Social Science & Medicine (1982)* 73, no. 6 (September 2011).

49. Anna Lowenhaupt Tsing, *Friction: An Ethnography of Global Connection* (Princeton, N.J.: Princeton University Press, 2005), 57.

50. Charis Thompson, *Making Parents: The Ontological Choreography of Reproductive Technologies* (Cambridge, Mass.: MIT Press, 2005); Herman Gray, "Subject(ed) to Recognition," *American Quarterly* 65, no. 4 (December 2013).

4. A DARK PAST IN PRESENT LIGHT

1. Irene Dankwa-Mullan and Yvonne T. Maddox, "Embarking on a Science Vision for Health Disparities Research," *American Journal of Public Health* 105, no. S3 (June 2015).

2. Mark Chaves and Lynn M. Higgins, "Comparing the Community Involvement of Black and White Congregations," *Journal for the Scientific Study of Religion* 31, no. 4 (December 1992); Linda M. Chatters, "Religion and Health: Public Health Research and Practice," *Annual Review of Public Health* 21 (2000); Jeff Levin, Linda M. Chatters, and Robert Joseph Taylor, "Religion, Health and Medicine in African Americans: Implications for Physicians," *Journal of the National Medical Association* 97, no. 2 (February 2005); Omar M. McRoberts, *Streets of Glory: Church and Community in a Black Urban Neighborhood* (Chicago: University of Chicago Press, 2005); S. Dodani and J. Z. Fields, "Implementation of the Fit Body and Soul, a Church-Based Life Style Program for Diabetes Prevention in High-Risk African Americans," *Diabetes Educator* 36, no. 3 (May 2010); Ian A. Gutierrez, Lucas J. Goodwin, Katherine Kirkinis, and Jacqueline S. Mattis, "Religious Socialization in African American Families: The Relative Influence of Par-

ents, Grandparents, and Siblings," *Journal of Family Psychology* 28, no. 6 (December 2014).

3. Ivor Lensworth Livingston, ed., *Handbook of Black American Health: The Mosaic of Conditions, Issues, Policies, and Prospects* (Westport, Conn.: Greenwood, 1994); Robert L. Hampton, Thomas P. Gullota, and Raymond L. Crowel, eds., *Handbook of African American Health* (New York: Guilford, 2010); Aletha Y. Akers, Selena Youmans, Stacy W. Lloyd, Dionne M. Smith, Bahby Banks, Connie Blumenthal, Tashuna Albritton, Arlinda Ellison, Giselle Corbie Smith, and Adaora A. Adimora, "Views of Young, Rural African Americans of the Role of Community Social Institutions in HIV Prevention," *Journal of Health Care for the Poor and Underserved* 21, 2 Suppl. (May 2010).

4. Sandra L. Barnes, "The Black Church Revisited: Toward a New Millennium DuBoisian Mode of Inquiry," *Sociology of Religion* 75, no. 4 (December 2014).

5. Chaves and Higgins, "Comparing the Community Involvement of Black and White Congregations"; Chatters, "Religion and Health"; Levin, Chatters, and Taylor, "Religion, Health, and Medicine in African Americans"; McRoberts, *Streets of Glory*; Dodani and Fields, "Implementation of the Fit Body and Soul"; Gutierrez et al., "Religious Socialization in African American Families."

6. Susan M. Reverby, *Examining Tuskegee: The Infamous Syphillis Study and Its Legacy* (Chapel Hill: University of North Carolina Press, 2009).

7. Alberto Corsín Jiménez, "Trust in Anthropology," *Anthropological Theory* 11, no. 2 (June 2011): 178.

8. Neighborhood /nābər͵hŏŏd/: a district, esp. one forming a community within a town or city.

9. John L. Jackson, *Harlemworld: Doing Race and Class in Contemporary Black America* (Chicago: University of Chicago Press, 2001); Robert J. Sampson and Patrick Sharkey, "Neighborhood Selection and the Social Reproduction of Concentrated Racial Inequality," *Demography* 45, no. 1 (February 2008); Mary Pattillo, *Black Picket Fences* (Chicago: University of Chicago Press, 2013).

10. Pierre Bourdieu and Loic Wacquant, "On the Cunning of Imperialist Reason," *Theory, Culture & Society* 16, no. 1 (February 1999); Michael J. Montoya, "Bioethnic Conscription: Genes, Race, and Mexicana/o Ethnicity in Diabetes Research," *Cultural Anthropology* 22, no. 1 (February 1, 2007): 94–128.

11. Clinical Research Center (CRC) is a pseudonym.

12. The Tuskegee Syphilis Study was conducted from 1932 to 1972 to observe the effects of untreated syphilis in a group of African American men. Although the study was discontinued after it was brought to public media

attention, researchers published the data in academic journals throughout the course of the project.

13. Darrell Whiteman, "One Significant Solution: How Anthropology Became the Number One Study for Evangelical Missionaries. Part II: Anthropology and Mission: The Incarnational Connection," *International Journal of Frontier Missions* 21, no. 1 (2004); Goldie S. Byrd, Christopher L. Edwards, Vinaya A. Kelkar, Ruth G. Phillips, Jennifer R. Byrd, Dora Som Pim-Pong, Takiyah D. Starks et al., "Recruiting Intergenerational African American Males for Biomedical Research Studies: A Major Research Challenge," *Journal of the National Medical Association* 103, no. 6 (June 2011).

14. Harriet A. Washington, *Medical Apartheid: The Dark History of Medical Experimentation on Black Americans from Colonial Times to the Present* (New York: Doubleday, 2006); Marci Kramish Campbell, Marlyn Allicock Hudson, Ken Resnicow, Natasha Blakeney, Amy Paxton, and Monica Baskin, "Church-Based Health Promotion Interventions: Evidence and Lessons Learned," *Annual Review of Public Health* 28 (2007); Ruha Benjamin, "Organized Ambivalence: When Sickle Cell Disease and Stem Cell Research Converge," *Ethnicity & Health* 16, no. 4–5 (August 2011); Joon-Ho Yu, Julia Crouch, Seema M. Jamal, Holly K. Tabor, and Michael J. Bamshad, "Attitudes of African Americans Toward Return of Results from Exome and Whole Genome Sequencing," *American Journal of Medical Genetics Part A* 161, no. 5 (April 2013).

15. St. Clair Drake, *The Redemption of Africa and Black Religion* (Chicago: Third World, 1970).

16. Alondra Nelson, *Body and Soul: The Black Panther Party and the Fight Against Medical Discrimination* (Minneapolis: University of Minnesota Press, 2011).

17. Nelson, *Body and Soul*; Gilbert King, *The Execution of Willie Francis: Race, Murder and the Search for Justice in the Jim Crow South* (New York: Civitas, 2009); Thomas J. Ward, *Black Physicians in the Jim Crow South* (Fayetteville: University of Arkansas Press, 2003).

18. See McRoberts, *Streets of Glory*; Kelly Brown Douglas and Ronald E. Hopson, "Understanding the Black Church: The Dynamics of Change," *Journal of Religious Thought* 56/57 (April 2001).

19. See Ingrid Overacker, *The African American Church Community in Rochester, New York, 1900–1940* (Rochester, N.Y.: University of Rochester Press, 1998). Ingrid Overacker examines the period before the massive influx of African Americans from the U.S. South and Caribbean into Rochester during the 1950s. Overacker writes a detailed history of four African American congregations in Rochester covering the first four decades of the twentieth century, of which Mt. Zion is one.

20. U.S. Census Bureau Administration and Customer Services Division,

"U.S. Census Bureau Publications—Census of Population and Housing," https://www.census.gov/prod/www/decennial.html.

21. R. D. G. Wadhwani, "Kodak, Fight and the Definition of Civil Rights in Rochester, New York 1966–1967," *Historian* 60, no. 1 (September 1997).

22. For an excellent visual history of the uprising, see *July '64*, directed by Carvin Eison, PBS, *Independent Lens,* February 14, 2006.

23. U.S. Census Bureau Administration and Customer Services Division, "Census of Population and Housing."

24. In late October 2011, Eastman Kodak Company announced that it had secured a $162 million cash loan to keep the company afloat. See Mike Spector and Dana Mattioli, "Eastman Kodak Seeks Rescue Financing," *Wall Street Journal* (October 25, 2011), https://www.wsj.com/articles/SB10001424052 9702047779045766516107071133324.

This was after the company had denied earlier reports that it was headed toward bankruptcy. See Andrew Martin and Michael J. de la Merced, "Kodak Hires Legal Adviser Amid Talk of Bankruptcy," *New York Times DealBook* (September 20, 2011), https://dealbook.nytimes.com/2011/09/30/kodak -hires-lawyers-weighs-bankruptcy-filing/; Julianne Pepitone, "Kodak Surges After Denying Bankruptcy Rumors," *CNNMoney* (October 3, 2011), money .cnn.com/2011/10/03/technology/kodak_bankruptcy_rumors/index.htm.

The Eastman Kodak Company eventually filed for bankruptcy in January 2012. See Michael J. de la Merced, "Eastman Kodak Files for Bankruptcy," *New York Times DealBook* (January 19, 2012), https://dealbook.nytimes.com/ 2012/01/19/eastman-kodak-files-for-bankruptcy/.

25. Jean M. Griffith, "Gentrification: Perspectives on the Return to the Central City," *Journal of Planning Literature* 11, no. 2 (November 1, 1996); Oren Yiftachel, "Planning and Social Control: Exploring the Dark Side," *Journal of Planning Literature* 12, no. 4 (May 1998); Oren Yiftachel, *Ethnocracy: Land and Identity Politics in Israel/Palestine* (Philadelphia: University of Pennsylvania Press, 2006).

26. For a more thorough treatment on the topic of reverse urban migration, see Isabel Wilkerson, *The Warmth of Other Suns: The Epic Story of America's Great Migration* (New York: Knopf Doubleday, 2010). This demographic phenomenon was confirmed by the 2010 U.S. Census, which showed a definite movement of African Americans from urban to rural areas as well as to the U.S. South.

27. U.S. Census Bureau, "American Community Survey Data Releases— 2012," https://www.census.gov/programs-surveys/acs/news/data-releases .html.

28. W. E. B. Du Bois and Isabel Eaton, *The Philadelphia Negro: A Social Study* (Philadelphia: University of Pennsylvania Press, 1899).

29. Barnes, "The Black Church Revisited."

30. Statistically, only one out of eleven African American boys in Rochester public schools who entered kindergarten in 2012 will graduate from high school. See Schott Foundation for Public Education, "The Urgency of Now: The Schott 50 State Report on Public Education and Black Males," (September 2012), http://schottfoundation.org/report/urgency-now-schott -50-state-report-public-education-and-black-males; Edward Doherty, "Poverty and the Concentration of Poverty in the Nine-County Rochester Area," Rochester Area Community Foundation (December 2013), https://www .actrochester.org/tinymce/source/2013%20Poverty%20Report.pdf.

31. The I Decide to Stop Diabetes Day at Church program formed part of a larger ADA initiative, Live EMPOWERED, aimed toward educating and increasing awareness in the African American community about diabetes. A similar initiative, Por tu Familia, (For Your Family) is geared toward the Latino community and another, Awakening the Spirit, seeks to address the diabetes epidemic among Native Americans, the group with the highest Type 2 diabetes rates in the United States. Upon a closer read, one can distinguish a difference in targeted emphasis between all three outreach efforts: The African American appeals to the self-agency of an individual "I" who "decides" to fight albeit alone, in contrast with the appeal to Latinos targeted not toward individuals, but to families. The Native American appeal speaks not to or about real individuals or families, but to a "spirit" that lives within a decimated remnant rendered invisible narratively, either as individuals or communities. See American Diabetes Association, *Launching a Movement to Stop Diabetes*, Annual Report (September 1, 2010), https://donations.diabetes .org/goh/generic/images/AnnualReport2009Online_090110.pdf.

32. Thornton Johnson et al. subsume racial, gender, education, and age concordances under the rubric "social concordance." Using an admittedly limited set of categories, the authors conclude that while patients associate high social concordance with increased patient satisfaction, notions of care, and willingness to refer friends to physicians, results showed higher concordance by race and gender, and less by age and education. See Rachel L. Johnson Thornton, Neil R. Powe, Debra Roter, and Lisa A. Cooper, "Patient–Physician Social Concordance, Medical Visit Communication and Patients' Perceptions of Health Care Quality," *Patient Education and Counseling* 85, no. 3 (December 2011).

33. See Aihwa Ong, "Making the Biopolitical Subject: Cambodian Immigrants, Refugee Medicine and Cultural Citizenship in California," *Social Science & Medicine (1982)* 40, no. 9 (May 1995).

34. Edouard Glissant, *Faulkner, Mississippi* (Chicago: University of Chicago Press, 1996), 29.

35. David S. FitzGerald and David Cook-Martín, "The Geopolitical Ori-

gins of the U.S. Immigration Act of 1965," *Migration Information Source*, February 5, 2014, https://www.migrationpolicy.org/article/geopolitical-origins-us-immigration-act-1965.

36. Presumably, there may well have been runaways with Caribbean backgrounds participating in the Underground Railroad. Also, the United Negro Movement Association (UNIA) begun by Marcus Garvey had a chapter in Western New York in the 1920s. The UNIA is credited with catalyzing West Indian immigration to the United States, especially New York. The flowering of the Harlem Renaissance, popularization of calypso music, and the genesis of the Nation of Islam, Rastafari, and the African Hebrew Israelites, among other groups, owe themselves to the circulation of people, ideas, and cultural forms of that period. See Jackson, *Harlemworld*; Claude McKay, *Harlem Shadows: The Poems of Claude McKay* (New York: Harcourt, Brace and Company, 1922). However, in terms of sheer numbers, I focus on the period 1952–1959. This historical lens does not avert our gaze from the unique black cultural habitus of the area, pre-1952, but, I argue, adds to the social complexity and cultural richness of the African American category in Rochester.

37. Centers for Disease Control and Prevention, *Number of Americans with Diabetes Projected to Double or Triple by 2050*, Press Release (Washington, D.C.: Division of News and Electronic Media, Office of Communication, October 22, 2010), http://www.cdc.gov/media/pressrel/2010/r101022.html.

38. American Diabetes Association, "The Economic Costs of Diabetes for 2017," *Diabetes Care* (March 21, 2018), https://care.diabetesjournals.org/content/early/2018/03/20/dci18-0007.

39. Jay S. Skyler, Richard Bergenstal, Robert O. Bonow, John Buse, Prakash Deedwania, Edwin A. M. Gale, Barbara V. Howard et al., "Intensive Glycemic Control and the Prevention of Cardiovascular Events: Implications of the ACCORD, ADVANCE, and VA Diabetes Trials: A Position Statement of the American Diabetes Association and a Scientific Statement of the American College of Cardiology Foundation and the American Heart Association," *Journal of the American College of Cardiology* 53, no. 3 (January 2009).

40. Felix Knauf and Peter S. Aronson, "ESRD as a Window into America's Cost Crisis in Health Care," *Journal of the American Society of Nephrology* 20, no. 10 (October 2009); Centers for Medicare & Medicaid Services, "ESRD—General Information," May 17, 2019, https://www.cms.gov/Medicare/End-Stage-Renal-Disease/ESRDGeneralInformation/index.html.

41. Andrew F. Stewart, "The U.S. Endocrinology Workforce Shortage: A Supply-Demand Mismatch," *Journal of Clinical Endocrinology and Metabolism* 93, no. 4 (April 2008): 1164.

42. Further, cosmetic surgery is not reimbursed by health insurance and is usually a straight cash transaction.

43. Stewart, "The U.S. Endocrinology Workforce Shortage," 1164.

44. Stewart, "The U.S. Endocrinology Workforce Shortage," 1164.

45. American Association of Clinical Endocrinologists, "About AACE," 2019, https://www.aace.com/about/about-american-association-clinical -endocrinologists.

46. With respect to women and gender, pharmacists, also allowed to become CDEs, are represented more equitably in this former male professional bastion. See Hedva Barenholtz Levy, "Women in Pharmacy 2006: A Good Match," *Annals of Pharmacotherapy* 40, no. 5 (May 2006).

47. Institute of Medicine (U.S.) Committee on Quality of Health Care in America, *Crossing the Quality Chasm: A New Health System for the 21st Century* (Washington, D.C.: National Academies Press, 2001).

48. Elizabeth B. Anderson, "Patient-Centeredness: A New Approach," *Nephrology News & Issues* 16, no. 12 (November 2002).

49. Shoumita Dasgupta, "Cultural Competency in the Medical Genetics Classroom: A Case Study for a Diverse Learning Community," *Medical Science Educator* 23, no. 2 (June 2013); Arno K. Kumagai and Monica L. Lypson, "Beyond Cultural Competence: Critical Consciousness, Social Justice, and Multicultural Education," *Academic Medicine: Journal of the Association of American Medical Colleges* 84, no. 6 (June 2009); Carla Boutin-Foster, Jordan C. Foster, and Lyuba Konopasek, "Viewpoint: Physician, Know Thyself: The Professional Culture of Medicine as a Framework for Teaching Cultural Competence," *Academic Medicine: Journal of the Association of American Medical Colleges* 83, no. 1 (January 2008); Sala Horowitz, "Cultural Competency Training in U.S. Medical Education: Treating Patients from Different Cultures," *Alternative and Complementary Therapies* 11, no. 6 (December 2005); L. Cooper-Patrick, J. J. Gallo, J. J. Gonzales, H. T. Vu, N. R. Powe, C. Nelson, and D. E. Ford, "Race, Gender, and Partnership in the Patient-Physician Relationship," *JAMA* 282, no. 6 (August 1999).

50. Horowitz, "Cultural Competency Training in U.S. Medical Education"; Cooper-Patrick et al., "Race, Gender, and Partnership in the Patient-Physician Relationship."

51. Jesse C. Crosson, Weiling Deng, Chantal Brazeau, Linda Boyd, and Maria Soto-Greene, "Evaluating the Effect of Cultural Competency Training on Medical Student Attitudes," *Family Medicine* 36, no. 3 (March 2004); Elyse R. Park, Maria B. J. Chun, Joseph R. Betancourt, Alexander R. Green, and Joel S. Weissman, "Measuring Residents' Perceived Preparedness and Skillfulness to Deliver Cross-cultural Care," *Journal of General Internal Medicine* 24, no. 9 (September 2009); Joel S. Weissman, Joseph Betancourt, Eric G. Campbell, Elyse R. Park, Minah Kim, Brian Clarridge, David Blumenthal, Karen C. Lee, and Angela W. Maina, "Resident Physicians' Preparedness to Provide Cross-Cultural Care," *JAMA* 294, no. 9 (September 2005).

52. Hospital Consumer Assessment of Healthcare Providers and Systems (HCAHPS), "HCAHPS Fact Sheet: November 2017," *CAHPS Hospital Survey,* November 28, 2017, https://www.hcahpsonline.org/globalassets/hcahps/facts/hcahps_fact_sheet_november_2017.pdf.

53. Sunil Kripalani, Jada Bussey-Jones, Marra G. Katz, and Inginia Genao, "A Prescription for Cultural Competence in Medical Education," *Journal of General Internal Medicine* 21, no. 10 (October 1, 2006): 1116–20.

54. Dorene F. Balmer, Christina L. Master, Boyd F. Richards, Janet R. Serwint, and Angelo P. Giardino, "An Ethnographic Study of Attending Rounds in General Paediatrics: Understanding the Ritual," *Medical Education* 44, no. 11 (November 2010).

55. Balmer et al., "An Ethnographic Study of Attending Rounds in General Paediatrics."

56. Elise Paradis, Myles Leslie, and Michael A. Gropper, "Interprofessional Rhetoric and Operational Realities: An Ethnographic Study of Rounds in Four Intensive Care Units," *Advances in Health Sciences Education* 21, no. 4 (October 1, 2016), https://doi.org/10.1007/s10459-015-9662-5.

57. Dorene F. Balmer, Christina L. Master, Boyd Richards, and Angelo P. Giardino, "Implicit Versus Explicit Curricula in General Pediatrics Education: Is There a Convergence?," *Pediatrics* 124, no. 2 (August 2009); Jann L. Murray-Garcia and Jorge A. Garcia, "The Institutional Context of Multicultural Education: What Is Your Institutional Curriculum?," *Academic Medicine: Journal of the Association of American Medical Colleges* 83, no. 7 (July 2008).

58. Steven J. Durning, Anthony R. Artino Jr, Louis N. Pangaro, Cees van der Vleuten, and Lambert Schuwirth, "Perspective: Redefining Context in the Clinical Encounter: Implications for Research and Training in Medical Education," *Academic Medicine: Journal of the Association of American Medical Colleges* 85, no. 5 (May 2010).

59. Joseph Gigante, "Direct Observation Medical Trainees," *Pediatrics and Therapeutics* 3 (2013); Stewart Babbott, "Commentary: Watching Closely at a Distance: Key Tensions in Supervising Resident Physicians," *Academic Medicine* 85, no. 9 (September 2010).

60. Désirée A. Lie, Elizabeth Lee-Rey, Art Gomez, Sylvia Bereknyei, and Clarence H. Braddock III, "Does Cultural Competency Training of Health Professionals Improve Patient Outcomes? A Systematic Review and Proposed Algorithm for Future Research," *Journal of General Internal Medicine* 26, no. 3 (March 2011).

61. Steven L. Kanter, "2011 Question of the Year," *Academic Medicine* 1, no. 1 (January 2011).

62. Janelle S. Taylor, "Confronting 'Culture' in Medicine's 'Culture of No Culture,'" *Academic Medicine* 78, no. 6 (June 2003).

63. Dawn W. Satterfield, Teresa Lofton, Jeannette E. May, Barbara A. Bowman, Ana Alfaro-Correa, Christopher Benjamin, and Melissa Stankus, "Learning from Listening: Common Concerns and Perceptions About Diabetes Prevention Among Diverse American Populations," *Journal of Public Health Management and Practice* 9, Supplement (November 2003); Institute of Medicine (U.S.) Committee on Understanding and Eliminating Racial and Ethnic Disparities in Health Care, *Unequal Treatment: Confronting Racial and Ethnic Disparities in Health Care* (Washington, D.C.: National Academies Press, 2002); Institute of Medicine (U.S.) Committee on Quality of Health Care in America, *Improving Medical Education: Enhancing the Behavioral and Social Science Content of Medical School Curricula* (Washington, D.C.: National Academies Press, 2004).

64. Cara S. Lesser, Catherine R. Lucey, Barry Egener, Clarence H. Braddock III, Stuart L. Linas, and Wendy Levinson, "A Behavioral and Systems View of Professionalism," *JAMA* 304, no. 24 (December 2010).

65. Jeffrey A. Katula, Mara Z. Vitolins, Erica L. Rosenberger, Caroline Blackwell, Mark A. Espeland, Michael S. Lawlor, W. Jack Rejeski, and David C. Goff, "Healthy Living Partnerships to Prevent Diabetes (HELP PD): Design and Methods," *Contemporary Clinical Trials* 31, no. 1 (January 2013).

66. Alison J. Scott and Robin Fretwell Wilson, "Social Determinants of Health among African Americans in a Rural Community in the Deep South: An Ecological Exploration," *Rural and Remote Health* 11, no. 1 (2011).

67. Katula et al., "Healthy Living Partnerships to Prevent Diabetes."

68. Satterfield et al., "Learning from Listening."

69. Southwest Rochester used to have five supermarkets to choose from: IGA on Genesee Street, Star Market on Jefferson Avenue, two supermarkets side-by-side on West Avenue (across from Unkle Moe's), and an A&P Market at Bullshead Plaza, later the site of a police substation.

70. In January 2020, the AADE changed its organizational name to the Association of Diabetes Care and Education Specialists (ADCES).

71. Charles L. Briggs, "Communicability, Racial Discourse, and Disease," *Annual Review of Anthropology* 34, no. 1 (2005): 269–91; Asif Agha, "Voice, Footing, Enregisterment," *Journal of Linguistic Anthropology* 15, no. 1 (2005); Charles L. Briggs and Daniel Hallin, "Biocommunicability: The Neoliberal Subject and Its Contradictions in News Coverage of Health Issues." *Social Text* 25 (December 1, 2007): 43–66.

72. Yam, *Dioscorea* sp., is a tropical root vegetable grown in Africa and the Caribbean. Outside of extreme South Florida, climatic conditions prevent its cultivation in the continental United States. Sweet potato, *Ipomea* sp., exists in many different varieties throughout the world. In the United States some sweet potatoes are called "yams," but all are actually sweet potatoes of the genus *Ipomea*.

73. For examples, see B. A. Leatherdale, R. K. Panesar, G. Singh, T. W. Atkins, C. J. Bailey, and A. H. Bignell, "Improvement in Glucose Tolerance due to *Momordica charantia* (Karela)," *British Medical Journal (Clinical Research Ed.)* 282, no. 6279 (June 1981); Muhammad Shoaib Akhtar, "Trial of *Momordica charantia linn* (Karela) Powder in Patients with Maturity-Onset Diabetes," *Journal of Pakistan Medical Association* 32, no. 4 (1982).

74. Gananath Obeyesekere, "The Impact of Ayurvedic Ideas on the Culture and the Individual in Sri Lanka," in *Asian Medical Systems: A Comparative Study*, ed. Leslie Charles (Berkeley: University of California Press, 1977); Dominik Wujastyk, *The Roots of Ayurveda: Selections from Sanskrit Medical Writings* (London: Penguin, 2003); Kenneth G. Zysk, *Religious Medicine: History and Evolution of Indian Medicine* (New York: Routledge, 2017).

75. Y. Monique Davis-Smith, John Mark Boltri, J. Paul Seale, Sylvia Shellenberger, Travis Blalock, and Brian Tobin, "Implementing a Diabetes Prevention Program in a Rural African-American Church," *Journal of the National Medical Association* 99, no. 4 (April 2007); Dodani and Fields, "Implementation of the Fit Body and Soul"; Yashika J. Watkins, Lauretta T. Quinn, Laurie Ruggiero, Michael T. Quinn, and Young-Ku Choi, "Spiritual and Religious Beliefs and Practices and Social Support's Relationship to Diabetes Self-Care Activities in African Americans," *Diabetes Educator* 39, no. 2 (March 2013); Gutierrez et al., "Religious Socialization in African American Families."

76. Fredrick C. Harris, *Something Within: Religion in African-America Political Activism* (Oxford: Oxford University Press, 1999).

77. See Bakari Kitwana, *The Hip-Hop Generation: Young Blacks and the Crisis in African-American Culture* (New York: Basic Books, 2002); Jordanna Matlon, "Creating Public Fictions: The Black Man as Producer and Consumer," *Black Scholar* 40, no. 3 (September 2010).

78. Brinton C. Clark, Ellie Grossman, Mary C. White, Joe Goldenson, and Jacqueline Peterson Tulsky, "Diabetes Care in the San Francisco County Jail," *American Journal of Public Health* 96, no. 9 (September 2006); Carolyn B. Sufrin, Amy M. Autry, Kathryn L. Harris, Joe Goldenson, and Jody E. Steinauer, "County Jail as a Novel Site for Obstetrics and Gynecology Resident Education," *Journal of Graduate Medical Education* 4, no. 3 (September 2012); American Diabetes Association, "Diabetes Management in Correctional Institutions," *Diabetes Care* 35, Supplement 1 (January 2012).

79. Byrd et al., "Recruiting Intergenerational African American Males."

80. Christopher J. L. Murray, Sandeep C. Kulkarni, Catherine Michaud, Niels Tomijima, Maria T. Bulzacchelli, Terrell J. Iandiorio, and Majid Ezzati, "Eight Americas: Investigating Mortality Disparities across Races, Counties, and Race-Counties in the United States," *PLOS Medicine* 3, no. 9 (September 2006).

81. John M. Klofas, Christopher Delaney, and Tisha Smith, "Strategic Approaches to Community Safety Initiative (SACSI) in Rochester, NY," Report submitted to the U.S. Department of Justice (November 2007), https://www.ncjrs.gov/pdffiles1/nij/grants/220488.pdf.

82. Schott Foundation for Public Education, "The Urgency of Now"; Doherty, "Poverty and the Concentration of Poverty in the Nine County Rochester Area."

83. Murray et al., "Eight Americas."

84. Veena Das and Ranendra K. Das, "Pharmaceuticals in Urban Ecologies," in *Global Pharmaceuticals: Ethics, Markets, Practices*, ed. Adriana Petryna, Andrew Lakoff, and Arthur Kleinman (Durham, N.C.: Duke University Press, 2006).

85. Jacob W. Gruber, "Ethnographic Salvage and the Shaping of Anthropology," *American Anthropologist* 72, no. 6 (December 1970); George W. Stocking Jr., *Race, Culture, and Evolution: Essays in the History of Anthropology* (Chicago: University of Chicago Press, 1968); J. D. Y. Peel, "For Who Hath Despised the Day of Small Things? Missionary Narratives and Historical Anthropology," *Comparative Studies in Society and History* 37, no. 3 (July 1995).

86. Bronislaw Malinowski, *Argonauts of the Western Pacific: An Account of Native Enterprise and Adventure in the Archipelagoes of Melanesian New Guinea* (London: Taylor & Francis, 2003); Edwin W. Smith, "Social Anthropology and Missionary Work," *International Review of Mission* 13, no. 4 (1924); E. E. Evans-Pritchard, *Witchcraft, Oracles and Magic among the Azande* (Oxford: Clarendon, 1937); Clifford Geertz, *Local Knowledge: Further Essays in Interpretive Anthropology* (New York: Basic Books, 1983).

87. Anderson, "Patient-Centeredness."

88. Malinowski, *Argonauts of the Western Pacific*; Claude Lévi-Strauss, *The Elementary Structures of Kinship* (Boston: Beacon, 1949); Marcel Mauss, *The Gift: The Form and Reason for Exchange in Archaic Societies* (New York: Routledge, 1954).

89. Jiménez, "Trust in Anthropology."

90. Jiménez, "Trust in Anthropology."

91. W. E. B. Du Bois, *The Negro Church: Report of a Social Study Made Under the Direction of Atlanta University; Together with the Proceedings of the Eighth Conference for the Study of the Negro Problems, Held at Atlanta University, May 26th, 1903* (Atlanta: University of Atlanta Press, 1903), ii.

92. Du Bois and Eaton, *The Philadelphia Negro*, 197.

5. THE ASCENSION OF THE BLACK MATRIARCH

1. See Frederic Golden, "The Race Is Over," *Time*, July 3, 2000, http://content.time.com/time/magazine/article/0,9171,997342,00.html.

2. Bryndis Yngvadottir, Daniel G Macarthur, Hanjun Jin, and Chris Tyler-Smith, "The Promise and Reality of Personal Genomics," *Genome Biology* 10, no. 9 (September 2009): 237.

3. See *Spiegel*, "SPIEGEL Interview with Craig Venter: 'We Have Learned Nothing from the Genome,'" *Spiegel Online*, July 29 2010, https://www.spiegel.de/international/world/spiegel-interview-with-craig-venter-we-have-learned-nothing-from-the-genome-a-709174.html.

4. Radoje Drmanac, Andrew B. Sparks, Matthew J. Callow, Aaron L. Halpern, Norman L. Burns, Bahram G. Kermani, Paolo Carnevali et al., "Human Genome Sequencing Using Unchained Base Reads on Self-Assembling DNA Nanoarrays," *Science* 327, no. 5961 (January 2010).

5. National Human Genome Research Institute, "Cost per Genome" (graphic), https://www.genome.gov/sites/default/files/inline-images/cost pergenome_2017.jpg. This graph shows the cost decline in genomic sequencing since June 2001. Note the sharp decline from mid-2007 to late 2011.

6. Kris A. Wetterstrand, "The Cost of Sequencing a Human Genome," *National Human Genome Research Institute* (2016), https://www.genome.gov/about-genomics/fact-sheets/Sequencing-Human-Genome-cost.

7. Sarah B. Ng, Kati J. Buckingham, Choli Lee, Abigail W. Bigham, Holly K. Tabor, Karin M. Dent, Chad D. Huff et al., "Exome Sequencing Identifies the Cause of a Mendelian Disorder," *Nature Genetics* 42, no. 1 (January 2010).

8. For example, see Rosa Fregel, Alejandra C. Ordóñez, Jonathan Santana-Cabrera, Vicente M. Cabrera, Javier Velasco-Vázquez, Verónica Alberto, Marco A. Moreno-Benítez et al., "Mitogenomes Illuminate the Origin and Migration Patterns of the Indigenous People of the Canary Islands," *PLOS ONE* 14, no. 3 (March 2019).

9. Melinda C. Mills and Charles Rahal, "A Scientometric Review of Genome-wide Association Studies," *Communications Biology* 2, no. 9 (January 2019).

10. Douglas C. Wallace, "Genetics: Mitochondrial DNA in Evolution and Disease," *Nature* 535, no. 7613 (July 2016).

11. Weihong Tang, Yuling Hong, Michael A. Province, Stephen S. Rich, Paul N. Hopkins, Donna K. Arnett, James S. Pankow, Michael B. Miller, and John H. Eckfeldt, "Familial Clustering for Features of the Metabolic Syndrome: The National Heart, Lung, and Blood Institute (NHLBI) Family Heart Study," *Diabetes Care* 29, no. 3 (March 2006).

12. Tang et al., "Familial Clustering for Features of the Metabolic Syndrome," 631.

13. Eleanor Wheeler and Ines Barroso, "Genome-Wide Association Studies and Type 2 Diabetes," *Briefings in Functional Genomics* 10, no. 2 (March 2011): 52.

14. For a more detailed account of the prospective polygenetic associations with T2D in the decade before 2017, see Peter M. Visscher, Naomi R. Wray, Qian Zhang, Pamela Sklar, Mark I. McCarthy, Matthew A. Brown, and Jian Yang, "10 Years of GWAS Discovery: Biology, Function, and Translation," *American Journal of Human Genetics* 101, no. 1 (July 6, 2017).

15. Rachel M. Sherman, Juliet Forman, Valentin Antonescu, Daniela Puiu, Michelle Daya, Nicholas Rafaels, Meher Preethi Boorgula et al., "Assembly of a Pan-genome from Deep Sequencing of 910 Humans of African Descent," *Nature Genetics* 51, no. 1 (January 2019).

16. The 1000 Genomes Project Consortium et al., "A Global Reference for Human Genetic Variation," *Nature* 526, no. 7571 (October 2015).

17. Mills and Rahal, "A Scientometric Review of Genome-wide Association Studies."

18. See Paul Rabinow, *French DNA: Trouble in Purgatory* (Chicago: University of Chicago Press, 1999); Jennifer A. Liu, "Aboriginal Fractions: Enumerating Identity in Taiwan," *Medical Anthropology* 31, no. 4 (2012).

19. Jacques Maquet, *Africanity: The Cultural Unity of Black Africa* (Oxford: Oxford University Press, 1972); L. S. Senghor, "The Study of African Man," *Mawazo* 1, no. 4 (1967).

20. Ricardo Morena Lima, Breno Silva de Abreu, Paulo Gentil, Tulio Cesar de Lima Lins, Dário Grattapaglia, Rinaldo Wellerson Pereira, and Ricardo Jacó de Oliveira, "Lack of Association between Vitamin D Receptor Genotypes and Haplotypes with Fat-Free Mass in Postmenopausal Brazilian Women," *Journals of Gerontology: Series A* 62, no. 9 (September 2007).

21. Harold A. McDougall, "Reconstructuring African American Cultural DNA: An Action Research Agenda for Howard University," *Howard Law Journal* 55 (2011–2012).

22. Didier Fassin, *When Bodies Remember: Experiences and Politics of AIDS in South Africa* (Berkeley: University of California Press, 2007); Stephan Palmié, *Africas of the Americas: Beyond the Search for Origins in the Study of Afro-Atlantic Religions* (Leiden, The Netherlands: Brill, 2008).

23. Palmié, *Africas of the Americas,* 57.

24. Catherine Bliss, *Race Decoded; The Genomic Fight for Social Justice* (Stanford, Calif.: Stanford University Press, 2012).

25. Wallace, "Genetics: Mitochondrial DNA in Evolution and Disease."

26. Vincent Brown, *The Reaper's Garden: Death and Power in the World of Atlantic Slavery* (Cambridge, Mass.: Harvard University Press, 2008).

27. See Charles N. Rotimi, Guanjie Chen, Adebowale A. Adeyemo, Paulette Furbert-Harris, Debra Parish-Gause, Jie Zhou, Kate Berg et al., "A Genome-Wide Search for Type 2 Diabetes Susceptibility Genes in West Africans: The Africa America Diabetes Mellitus (AADM) Study," *Diabetes* 53,

no. 3 (March 2004); Rasika Ann Mathias, Margaret A. Taub, Christopher R. Gignoux, Wenqing Fu, Shaila Musharoff, Timothy D. O'Connor, Candelaria Vergara et al., "A Continuum of Admixture in the Western Hemisphere Revealed by the African Diaspora Genome," *Nature Communications* 7 (October 11, 2016).

28. Andrew Adey, Joshua N. Burton, Jacob O. Kitzman, Joseph B. Hiatt, Alexandra P. Lewis, Beth K. Martin, Ruolan Qiu, Choli Lee, and Jay Shendure, "The Haplotype-Resolved Genome and Epigenome of the Aneuploid HeLa Cancer Cell Line," *Nature* 500, no. 7461 (August 2013).

29. Jonathan J. M. Landry, Paul Theodor Pyl, Tobias Rausch, Thomas Zichner, Manu M. Tekkedil, Adrian M. Stütz, Anna Jauch et al., "The Genomic and Transcriptomic Landscape of a HeLa Cell Line," *G3: Genes, Genomes, Genetics* 3, no. 8 (August 1, 2013).

30. Hannah Landecker, "Immortality, In Vitro: A History of the HeLa Cell Line." In *Biotechnology and Culture: Bodies, Anxieties, Ethics,* ed. Paul Brodwin (Bloomington: Indiana University Press, 2000); Rebecca Skloot, *The Immortal Life of Henrietta Lacks* (New York: Broadway Paperbacks, 2011).

31. National Institutes of Health, "NIH, Lacks Family Reach Understanding to Share Genomic Data of HeLa Cells," August 7, 2013, https://www.nih.gov/news-events/news-releases/nih-lacks-family-reach-understanding-share-genomic-data-hela-cells.

32. Karla F. C. Holloway, *Private Bodies, Public Texts: Race, Gender, and a Cultural Bioethics* (Durham, N.C.: Duke University Press, 2011), 7.

33. Max Weber, "Remarks on Technology and Culture," *Theory, Culture & Society* 22, no. 4 (August 2005 [1910]): 27.

34. See Kathy L. Hudson, "Data Sharing and the HeLa Genome Sequence," *69th Meeting of the National Advisory Council for Human Genome Research* (Rockville, Md.: National Human Genome Research Institute, September 9–10, 2013), https://www.genome.gov/Pages/About/NACHGR/NACHGRMeetingSummaries/Sept2013CouncilMinutes.pdf.

35. Kathy L. Hudson and Francis S. Collins, "Bringing the Common Rule into the 21st Century," *New England Journal of Medicine* 373, no. 24 (December 10, 2015).

36. It should be noted that the time between the Belmont Report's 1979 release and recommendations until the implementation of the Common Rule in 1992 spanned three successive Republican administrations, while the 2013 changes to the Common Rule occurred during the Obama administration.

37. Office of the Secretary, National Commission for the Protection of Human Subjects of Biomedical and Behavioral Research, *The Belmont Report: Ethical Principles and Guidelines for the Protection of Human Subjects of Research* (Washington, D.C.: Department of Health, Education, and Welfare,

April 18, 1979). See also, Todd W. Rice, "The Historical, Ethical, and Legal Background of Human-Subjects Research," *Respiratory Care* 53, no. 10 (October 2008).

38. Office of the Secretary, National Commission for the Protection of Human Subjects of Biomedical and Behavioral Research, *The Belmont Report.*

39. Leroy Walters, "Patricia King: Oral History of the Belmont Report and the National Commission for the Protection of Human Subjects of Biomedical and Behavioral Research," U.S. Department of Health and Human Services, Office for Human Research Protections, https://www.hhs.gov/ohrp/education-and-outreach/luminaries-lecture-series/belmont-report-25th-anniversary-interview-pking/index.html. For a larger treatment of the Tuskegee Study, see Susan M. Reverby, *Examining Tuskegee: The Infamous Syphilis Study and Its Legacy* (Chapel Hill: University of North Carolina Press, 2009).

40. Office of the Secretary, National Commission for the Protection of Human Subjects of Biomedical and Behavioral Research, *The Belmont Report.*

41. Adriana Petryna, "Clinical Trials Offshored: On Private Sector Science and Public Health," *BioSocieties* 2, no. 1 (March 2007). For a fuller treatment, see Adriana Petryna, *When Experiments Travel: Clinical Trials and the Global Search for Human Subjects* (Princeton, N.J.: Princeton University Press, 2009).

42. Michel Foucault, *The Birth of the Clinic: An Archaeology of Medical Perception* (London: Routledge Classics, 2003).

43. Deborah R. Gordon, "Tenacious Assumptions of Western Medicine," in *Biomedicine Examined,* ed. Deborah R. Gordon and Margaret Lock (Dordrecht: Springer Netherlands, [1988] 2012). Öncel Naldemirci, Doris Lydahl, Nicky Britten, Mark Elam, Lucy Moore, and Axel Wolf, "Tenacious Assumptions of Person-Centred Care?: Exploring Tensions and Variations in Practice," *Health* 22, no. 1 (January 1, 2018).

44. David Armstrong, *Political Anatomy of the Body: Medical Knowledge in Britain in the Twentieth Century* (Cambridge: Cambridge University Press, 1983).

45. Jacob Metcalf, "Big Data Analytics and Revision of the Common Rule," *Communications of the ACM* 59, no. 7 (July 2016).

46. Phoebe Friesen, Lisa Kearns, Barbara Redman, and Arthur L. Caplan, "Rethinking the Belmont Report?," *American Journal of Bioethics* 17, no. 7 (July 2017).

47. Sara Chandros Hull and David R. Wilson, "Beyond Belmont: Ensuring Respect for AI/AN Communities through Tribal IRBs, Laws, and Policies," *American Journal of Bioethics* 17, no. 7 (July 2017).

48. Hilary Beckles, *Centering Woman: Gender Discourses in Caribbean Slave*

Society (Kingston, Jamaica: Ian Randle, 1999); Edith Clarke, *My Mother Who Fathered Me: A Study of the Families in Three Selected Communities of Jamaica* (Kingston, Jamaica: University of the West Indies Press, 1999); Edward Franklin Frazier, *The Negro Family in the United States* (Notre Dame, Ind.: University of Notre Dame Press, 1939); Herbert H. Hyman and John Shelton Reed, "'Black Matriarchy' Reconsidered: Evidence From Secondary Analysis of Sample Surveys," *Public Opinion Quarterly* 33, no. 3 (1969); Daniel Patrick Moynihan, *The Negro Family: The Case for National Action* (Washington, D.C.: U.S. Government Printing Office, 1965); Raymond T. Smith, *The Negro Family in British Guiana: Family Structure and Social Status in the Villages* (New York: Routledge, [1956] 1998); Raymond T. Smith, *Kinship and Class in the West Indies: A Genealogical Study of Jamaica and Guyana* (Cambridge: Cambridge University Press, 1988); Raymond T. Smith, *The Matrifocal Family: Power, Pluralism, and Politics* (New York: Routledge, 1996).

49. J. Lorand Matory, *Black Atlantic Religion: Tradition, Transnationalism, and Matriarchy in the Afro-Brazilian Candomble* (Princeton, N.J.: Princeton University Press, 2005); Peggy Reeves Sanday, "Matriarchy as a Sociocultural Form: An Old Debate in a New Light," *16th Congress of the Indo-Pacific Prehistory Association*, July 1–7, 1998, https://web.sas.upenn.edu/psanday/articles/selected-articles/matriarchy-as-a-sociocultural-form-an-old-debate-in-a-new-light/.

50. Lisa H. Weasel, "Feminist Intersections in Science: Race, Gender and Sexuality through the Microscope," *Hypatia* 19, no. 1 (February 2004): 189; see Landecker, "Immortality, In Vitro."

51. Bliss, *Race Decoded*.

52. Keith Wailoo, Alondra Nelson, and Catherin Lee, eds., *Genetics and the Unsettled Past: The Collision of DNA, Race, and History* (New Brunswick, N.J.: Rutgers University Press, 2012).

53. For two separate accounts charting the scholarly arc of this discussion spanning a ten-year period, see Amade M'charek, "The Mitochondrial Eve of Modern Genetics: Of Peoples and Genomes, or the Routinization of Race," *Science as Culture* 14, no. 2 (June 2005); Venla Oikkonen, "Mitochondrial Eve and the Affective Politics of Human Ancestry: Winner of the 2015 Catharine Stimpson Prize for Outstanding Feminist Scholarship," *Signs: Journal of Women in Culture and Society* 40, no. 3 (March 2015): 748.

54. Anne Fausto-Sterling, "The Bare Bones of Sex: Part 1—Sex and Gender," *Signs: Journal of Women in Culture and Society* 30, no. 2 (January 2005); Oikkonen, "Mitochondrial Eve and the Affective Politics of Human Ancestry."

55. Ralph Linton, *The Study of Man: An Introduction* (New York: D. Appleton-Century, 1936); Kingsley Davis, *Human Society* (New York:

Macmillan, 1950); Talcott Parsons, "Equality and Inequality in Modern Society, or Social Stratification Revisited," *Sociological Inquiry* 40, no. 2 (April 1970); Barbara F. Reskin, "Including Mechanisms in Our Models of Ascriptive Inequality," in *Handbook of Employment Discrimination Research: Rights and Realities,* ed. Laura Beth Nielsen and Robert L. Nelson (New York: Springer, 2005); Barbara F. Reskin and Debra Branch McBrier, "Why Not Ascription? Organizations' Employment of Male and Female Managers," *American Sociological Review* 65, no. 2 (April 2000).

56. Not all peers inherit their predecessors' social status. Only dukes, earls, viscounts, marquesses, and barons may inherit peerage titles intergenerationally. See Debretts London 1769, *The Essential Guide to the Peerage* (London: Debretts, Limited, 2019), https://www.debretts.com/expertise/essential-guide-to-the-peerage/.

57. Sanday, "Matriarchy as a Sociocultural Form."

58. Smith, *The Matrifocal Family.*

59. Sanday, "Matriarchy as a Sociocultural Form."

60. Bridget Brereton, *Race Relations in Colonial Trinidad 1870–1900* (Cambridge: Cambridge University Press, 2002).

61. Hortense J. Spillers, "Mama's Baby, Papa's Maybe: An American Grammar Book," *Diacritics* 17, no. 2 (1987): 64.

62. Over 80,000 of the nearly 138,000 articles on HeLa by June 2019 were published after 2010; 32,500 of the nearly 60,000 NIH grants for HeLa research were awarded between 2010 and 2019, see PubMed Central, National Institutes of Health, National Library of Medicine, search for "HeLa" with filter 01/01/2010–06/31/2019, https://www.ncbi.nlm.nih.gov/pmc.

63. Ewen Callaway, "Deal Done over HeLa Cell Line," *Nature News* 500, no. 7461 (August 2013): 133.

64. Saidiya Hartman, *Lose Your Mother: A Journey Along the Atlantic Slave Route* (London: Macmillan, 2007), 233.

65. Richard Hyland, "Gift and Danger," *Journal of Classical Sociology* 14, no. 1 (February 1, 2014): 52.

66. Joan W. Scott, "Gender: A Useful Category of Historical Analysis," *American Historical Review* 91, no. 5 (1986): 1068.

67. Susan Reverby uncovered official records of U.S. government syphilis experiments conducted on prisoners in Guatemala during the 1940s. These offshore experiments sought to avoid the seemingly onerous ethical restrictions that officials argued prevented more aggressive research domestically in the Tuskegee Syphilis Study. See Susan M. Reverby, "Ethical Failures and History Lessons: The U.S. Public Health Service Research Studies in Tuskegee and Guatemala," *Public Health Reviews* 34, no. 1 (2012): 1–18.

68. Annemarie Mol, *The Logic of Care: Health and the Problem of Patient Choice* (New York: Routledge, 2008).

CONCLUSION

1. Georges Canguilhem, *On the Normal and the Pathological* (Dordrecht, The Netherlands: D. Reidel, 1978).

2. Similarly, Sangaramoorthy demonstrated how HIV risk-prevention and treatment programs geared toward the Haitian community in South Florida faced political, racial, and cultural challenges in formulating effective care for a marginalized and stigmatized community. Thurka Sangaramoorthy, *Treating AIDS: Politics of Difference, Paradox of Prevention* (New Brunswick, N.J.: Rutgers University Press, 2014).

3. Cf. Rogers Brubaker, *Ethnicity without Groups* (Cambridge, Mass.: Harvard University Press, 2004).

4. Deborah A. Bolnick, Duana Fullwiley, Troy Duster, Richard S. Cooper, Joan H. Fujimura, Jonathan Kahn, Jay S. Kaufman et al. "The Science and Business of Genetic Ancestry Testing," *Science* 318, no. 5849 (October 19, 2007): 399–400.

5. Paul Rabinow, *Making PCR: A Story of Biotechnology* (Chicago: University of Chicago Press, 1996).

6. Andrew Adey, Joshua N. Burton, Jacob O. Kitzman, Joseph B. Hiatt, Alexandra P. Lewis, Beth K. Martin, Ruolan Qiu, Choli Lee, and Jay Shendure, "The Haplotype-Resolved Genome and Epigenome of the Aneuploid HeLa Cancer Cell Line," *Nature* 500, no. 7461 (August 8, 2013): 207–11.

7. See Robert Mitchell and Catherine Waldby, "National Biobanks: Clinical Labor, Risk Production, and the Creation of Biovalue," *Science, Technology, & Human Values* 35, no. 3 (May 2010).

8. Melanie White and Alan Hunt, "Citizenship: Care of the Self, Character and Personality," *Citizenship Studies* 4, no. 2 (June 2000).

9. Michel de Certeau, *The Practice of Everyday Life* (Berkeley: University of California Press, 1984), 149.

10. Nancy Scheper-Hughes and Margaret Lock, "The Mindful Body: A Prolegomenon to Future Work in Medical Anthropology," *Medical Anthropology Quarterly* 1, no. 1 (March 1987); Annemarie Mol, *The Body Multiple: Ontology in Medical Practice* (Durham, N.C.: Duke University Press, 2002).

11. Cf. Joseph Dumit, "Drugs for Life," *Molecular Interventions* 2, no. 3 (2002).

12. Nikolas Rose, *The Politics of Life Itself: Biomedicine, Power, and Subjectivity in the Twenty-First Century* (Princeton, N.J.: Princeton University Press, 2007).

13. Cf. Vincanne Adams, Suellen Miller, Sienna Craig, Arlene Samen, Nyima, Sonam, Droyoung, Lhakpen, and Michael Varner, "The Challenge of Cross-Cultural Clinical Trials Research: Case Report from the Tibetan Autonomous Region, People's Republic of China," *Medical Anthropology*

Quarterly 19, no. 3 (September 2005). For the authors, even the notion of "research" required a translational toolkit. Traditional Tibetan medical indices of therapeutic effectiveness do not tend to separate healing dynamics from social and/or religious processes. As with racial classification, biomedical notions of therapeutic efficacy in Tibet were predicated upon statistical determinations of risk generated from essentialized patient populations, rather than a focus upon the individual. It located efficacy in the patient through the statistical mean, leaving no room for those statistical outliers representing real human, medical, and ethnographic "fact." In this regard, traditional Tibetan medical epistemology would assume these patient-outliers as examples of their system's rules, not exceptions (pp. 276–78). I attend the same concerned theoretical and methodological focus in arguing for ethnographic ontologies of the statistical outlier within the contemporary U.S. Type 2 diabetic field.

14. Jeremy A. Greene, *Prescribing by Numbers: Drugs and the Definition of Disease* (Baltimore, Md.: Johns Hopkins University Press, 2007).

15. Charis Thompson, "Race Science," *Theory, Culture, and Society* 23, no. 2–3, (May 1, 2006): 547.

16. Cf. João Biehl, *Vita: Life in a Zone of Social Abandonment* (Berkeley: University of California Press, 2013).

17. Biehl, *Vita*; Michel S. Laguerre, *Minoritized Space: An Inquiry into the Spatial Order of Things* (Berkeley: Institute of Governmental Studies Press, 1999).

18. Ruha Benjamin, "Organized Ambivalence: When Sickle Cell Disease and Stem Cell Research Converge," *Ethnicity & Health* 16, no. 4–5 (August 1, 2011): 447–63.

19. Talal Asad, *Anthropology and the Colonial Encounter* (New York: Humanities Press, 1973), 16.

20. Asad, *Anthropology and the Colonial Encounter,* 17–18.

21. Asad, *Anthropology and the Colonial Encounter,* 18–19.

22. Asad, *Anthropology and the Colonial Encounter,* 104.

23. Trouillot questioned, through Latour, the hegemonic truth claims of the modernity narrative itself. See Michel-Rolph Trouillot, *Global Transformations: Anthropology and the Modern World* (New York: Palgrave Macmillan, 2003), 45–46. Cf. Bruno Latour, *We Have Never Been Modern,* trans. Catherine Porter (Cambridge, Mass.: Harvard University Press, 2012).

24. David Barton Smith, "Racial and Ethnic Health Disparities and the Unfinished Civil Rights Agenda," *Health Affairs* 24, no. 2 (March 2005); Mary-Jo DelVecchio-Good, Byron J. Good, and Anne E. Becker, "The Culture of Medicine and Racial, Ethnic and Class Disparities in Health Care," in *Unequal Treatment: Confronting Racial and Ethnic Disparities in Health Care,* ed. Institute of Medicine (U.S.) Committee on Understanding and Eliminat-

ing Racial and Ethnic Disparities in Health Care, Brian D. Smedley, Adrienne Y. Stith, and Alan R. Nelson (Washington, D.C.: National Academies Press, 2003). In the illustrative case of Baltimore, see Rebecca Skloot, *The Immortal Life of Henrietta Lacks* (New York: Broadway Paperbacks, 2011).

25. Cf. Veena Das and Ranendra Das, "Pharmaceuticals in Urban Ecologies: The Register of the Local," in *Global Pharmaceuticals: Ethics, Markets, Practices*, ed. Adriana Petryna, Andrew Lakoff, and Arthur Kleinman (Durham, N.C.: Duke University Press, 2006).

26. Ashanté M. Reese, *Black Food Geographies: Race, Self-Reliance, and Food Access in Washington, D.C.* (Chapel Hill: University of North Carolina Press, 2018).

27. Niklas Luhmann, *Observations on Modernity* (Palo Alto, Calif.: Stanford University Press, 1998).

28. Marcel Mauss, *The Gift: The Form and Reason for Exchange in Archaic Societies* (New York: Routledge, 1954), 82.

29. Mauss, *The Gift*, 82–83.

30. Max Weber, "Remarks on Technology and Culture," *Theory, Culture & Society* 22, no. 4 (August 1, 2005): 23–38.

31. Hortense J. Spillers, "Mama's Baby, Papa's Maybe: An American Grammar Book," *Diacritics* 17, no. 2 (1987): 74.

32. Richard Hyland, "Gift and Danger," *Journal of Classical Sociology* 14, no. 1 (February 1, 2014): 50.

33. This was evidenced by the example of Tuskegee Institute's plans to open a bioethics center despite the fact that communities in the area around the university continue to suffer from a lack of access to basic quality medical care. See Jenny Reardon, *The Postgenomic Condition* (Chicago: University of Chicago Press, 2017).

34. Rose, *The Politics of Life Itself*; J.-A. Mbembé and Libby Meintjes, "Necropolitics," *Public Culture* 15, no. 1 (March 2003).

35. Harriet A. Washington, *Medical Apartheid: The Dark History of Medical Experimentation on Black Americans from Colonial Times to the Present* (New York: Doubleday, 2006).

36. Mary-Jo del Vecchio Good, Byron J. Good, Cynthia Schaffer, and Stuart E. Lind, "American Oncology and the Discourse on Hope," *Culture, Medicine, and Psychiatry* 14, no. 1 (March 1990).

37. See Gayatri Spivak, "Can the Subaltern Speak?," in *Can the Subaltern Speak? Reflections on the History of an Idea*, ed. Rosalind Morris (New York: Columbia University Press, 2010); Timothy Mitchell, "Can the Mosquito Speak?," in *Rule of Experts: Egypt, Techno-Politics, Modernity* (Berkeley: University of California Press, 2002); Denise Ferreira Da Silva, "'Bahia Pêlo Negro': Can the Subaltern (Subject of Raciality) Speak?," *Ethnicities* 5, no. 3 (September 2005).

38. John L. Jackson, *Real Black: Adventures in Racial Sincerity* (Chicago: University of Chicago Press, 2005).

39. Jackson, *Real Black*.

40. Jackson, *Real Black*, 15.

41. Kaushik Sunder Rajan, "Subjects of Speculation: Emergent Life Sciences and Market Logics in the United States and India," *American Anthropologist* 107, no. 1 (March 2005): 24.

42. See, Ashis Nandy, *Science as a Reason of State* (Oxford: Oxford University Press, 1988); Charis Thompson, *Making Parents: The Ontological Choreography of Reproductive Technologies* (Cambridge, Mass.: MIT Press, 2005).

Index

Abrego, Dr. (pseudonym), 60, 61
Action in Diabetes and Vascular Disease—Preterax and Diamicron Modified Release Controlled Evaluation (ADVANCE), 46, 47–49, 138
Action to Control Cardiovascular Risk in Diabetes (ACCORD), 47–49, 138
Adey, Andrew, 115
admixture: Africanicity and, 109–13, 114; definition of, 157; genetic technologies and, 13; genomic research and, 20, 102, 105, 106; matriarchy and, 123–24, 130; risk and, 15
adult-onset diabetes, 24. *See also* Type 2 diabetes (T2D)
Africa, sub-Saharan, xviii, 15, 20–21, 102, 104, 110–14, 117, 120–21, 124, 128, 148, 157
African American populations: admixture and, 114; biovalue of, 145–46; DRS and, 145; GWAS and, 106; health disparities among, 76; matriarchy and, 121; Mt. Zion and, 80–81, 182n19; outreach efforts to, 94; recruitment of, 69–70, 76–77, 78, 94–96, 120, 184n31; risk and, 53; in Rochester, 82, 184n30; soldiers, 35–36; Tethys

BioSciences and, 54–59, 139; in trials, 128–29; as volunteers, 142; wanting African American researchers' involvement, 136
African Americans: as aliens, 10, 165n33; author's use of term, 8, 22; as property, 34
African-descent populations: clinical research and, 15; diversity science and, 106; DNA from, 109; and genetic diversity, 135; genomic sampling recruitment of, 21; outreach to, 14, 73; as population samples, 136; recruitment of, 19, 141; slave societies and, 114; as a social group, 75–76; trust and, 98
Africanicity, 111, 112, 114, 148, 157
African populations, 35, 53, 170n29, 176n9
African retentions, 12
Africoid, 111
Afro-Brazilian populations, 112
Afro-Caribbean populations, 36, 53, 106, 112, 176n9
Afro-Creole populations, 9, 52, 58, 121
Afro-French Creole ethnicity, xi, 9
Alameda County Department of Public Health, xvi, 1, 54, 87, 149
Alzheimer's disease, 37, 82, 83, 113
"America" (Blake), 33, 34

James Doucet-Battle is assistant professor in the Department of Sociology at the University of California, Santa Cruz.